PRK

The Past, Present, and Future of Surface Ablation

PRK

The Past, Present, and Future of Surface Ablation

Lucio Buratto, MD

Steven G. Slade, MD, FACS

Sebastiano Serrao, MD, PhD

Marco Lombardo, MD, PhD

CRC Press
Taylor & Francis Group
Boca Raton London New York

CRC Press is an imprint of the
Taylor & Francis Group, an **informa** business

First published 2012 by SLACK Incorporated

Published 2024 by CRC Press
2385 NW Executive Center Drive, Suite 320, Boca Raton FL 33431

and by CRC Press
4 Park Square, Milton Park, Abingdon, Oxon, OX14 4RN

CRC Press is an imprint of Taylor & Francis Group, LLC

Buratto, Lucio.
PRK : past, present, and future / Lucio Buratto, Stephen G. Slade.
p. ; cm.
Photorefractive keratectomy
Includes bibliographical references and index.
ISBN 978-1-61711-043-6 (alk. paper)
1. Cornea--Laser surgery. 2. LASIK (Eye surgery) I. Slade, Stephen, 1953- II. Title. III. Title: Photorefractive keratectomy.
[DNLM: 1. Photorefractive Keratectomy--methods. 2. Cornea--surgery. 3. Keratomileusis, Laser In Situ. WW 340]
RE336.B87 2012
617.7'190598--dc23

2011029800

ISBN: 9781617110436 (hbk)
ISBN: 9781003525950 (ebk)

DOI: 10.1201/9781003525950

Dedications

To my brother Quinzio.
Lucio Buratto, MD

To Cyndi, Rachael, Jacqueline, and Sam.
Gwen too!
Steven G. Slade, MD, FACS

To my family, a real treasure.
Sebastiano Serrao, MD, PhD

To my brothers and friends.
Marco Lombardo, MD, PhD

Contents

Acknowledgments

First of all, I would like to thank Sebastiano Serrao and Marco Lombardo for their invaluable and scrupulous commitment which was fundamental for the completion of this book.
My thanks also to all of the collaborators who were part of this project. They were invited to participate because they are expert in their fields—they are gifted with renowned professional competence and also an astonishing ability to write clearly to enthusiastically encourage their colleagues through their professional knowledge.
I would like to thank Steve Slade—I am grateful for his patience, his readiness to help, and his unfailing good mood.
My thanks to the staff of Medicongress for all their invaluable organization and operative support.

Lucio Buratto, MD

About the Authors

Lucio Buratto, MD is considered a leading international expert in cataract and myopia surgery. He is a pioneer in IOL implantation; in phacoemulsification; and in laser techniques for myopia, astigmatism, and hyperopia. Since 1980, Dr. Buratto has organized and presided over 47 updating congresses on cataract and glaucoma surgery and on laser therapy. He also organized 54 practical courses for the teaching of eye surgery and served as spokesman and teacher in 386 courses and congresses.

In 1989, Dr. Buratto presented and was the world's first surgeon to use the excimer laser for intrastromal keratomileusis, and concurrently also started to treat low myopia using PRK techniques. In 1996, he was the world's first surgeon to use the new technique called "Down-Up LASIK," which improved the LASIK procedure for the correction of myopia. For teaching purposes, Dr. Buratto has performed surgical operations during live surgery sessions for more than 200 international and Italian congresses; performed surgery during satellite broadcasts to 54 countries in 4 different continents; and designed and produced 136 instruments for ocular surgery.

Dr. Buratto has written over 125 scientific publications and 53 monographs dedicated to ophthalmic surgery and has received several awards, including Maestro of Italian Ophthalmology with Medal of Merit (1998); Barraquer, during the International Congress of the American Academy (2000); Binkhorst Lecture during the XXII Annual Meeting, Paris (2004); and Fyodorov Medal at the HSIOIRS meeting, Athens (2006).

Since 2007, Dr. Buratto has been Honorary President of AISO (Italian Academy of Ophthalmological Sciences) and past president of AICCER (Italian Association of Cataract and Refractive Surgery). Presently, he is the director of Centro Ambrosiano Oftalmico (Ophthalmic Microsurgery Center), and practices at his private profession in Milan.

Stephen G. Slade, MD, FACS is a native Houstonian and is in private practice in Houston, TX. He graduated Summa Cum Laude and Phi Beta Kappa from the University of Texas at Austin and the University of Texas Medical School with a final elective year spent at Guy's Hospital, London, UK. He completed a residency at the LSU Eye Center in New Orleans, LA and fellowships in cataract and corneal surgery at Baylor College of Medicine in Houston and in New York, NY on Project ORBIS.

Dr. Slade is a fellow of the American Academy of Ophthalmology and the American College of Surgeons. He is an active teacher of surgical techniques and has taught and certified over 8,000 surgeons in LASIK and lamellar refractive surgery. Several hundred have chosen him for their own surgery. Dr. Slade is also an active researcher and has served as medical monitor for several new technologies, including laser cataract surgery, wavefront LASIK, ICLs, femtosecond lasers, keratophakia and accommodating IOLs. He has the nation's longest experience in LASIK (along with Stephen Brint, MD), femtosecond laser LASIK, accommodating IOLs, and femtosecond laser cataract surgery.

Dr. Slade has received numerous awards including 18 named lectures, Refractive Surgeon of the Year, two China Service Medals, the Lans Award, the Casebeer Award, and the 2007 Barraquer Award. Dr. Slade was selected by his peers for "Best Doctors," "Texas Super Doctors," and "Best Doctors in America" and has received the Senior Honor Award of the American Academy of Ophthalmology. He is a regular presenter at medical meetings and has received several "Best Speaker" awards and has twice won First Place at the American Society of Cataract and Refractive Surgery Film Festival. He is on several editorial boards, including the Journal of Refractive Surgery, and serves as Chief Medical Editor of Cataract and Refractive Surgery Today as well as President of the American College of Ophthalmic Surgery.

Dr. Slade has produced many articles and book chapters, holds 5 patents or patents pending in the field, and has authored or co-authored 8 textbooks on ophthalmic surgery. Dr. Slade has appeared on ABC, CBS, CNN, NYT, WSJ and was the featured surgeon on the Emmy award-winning PBS documentary "20/10 by 2010?" narrated by Walter Chronkite.

Sebastiano Serrao, MD, PhD graduated with a degree in medicine and surgery in 1992 then continued on to specialize in ophthalmology in 1996. In 2004, he completed his PhD in ophthalmology and surgical correction of refractive defects at the University of Padua, Italy. Dr. Serrao has trained at Moorfields Eye Hospital, London (1996), Revision Eye Center, Ohio (2000), and the Wilmer Eye Institute at the Johns Hopkins Hospital, Maryland (2002). Dr. Serrao is the founder and director of the refractive and cataract Centre "Serraolaser" in Rome, Italy and the author of more than 25 peer-reviewed papers. He has been working as a researcher at IRCCS Fondazione G. B. Bietti in Rome, Italy since January 2010.

Marco Lombardo, MD, PhD graduated summa cum laude with a degree in medicine and surgery in 1999 from the University of Rome "La Sapienza." He specialized in ophthalmology in 2003 and graduated summa cum laude from the Catholic University of Rome. He earned his PhD in Biomedical and Computer Engineering in 2007. Dr. Lombardo's research fields of interest are corneal biomechanics and human optics and innovation technologies in ophthalmology, including adaptive optics and nano-targeted drug delivery. He is the author of more than 25 peer-reviewed papers and serves on a regular basis as a reviewer for 9 scientific journals. Dr. Lombardo has been working as a researcher at IRCCS Fondazione G. B. Bietti in Rome, Italy since January 2010.

Contributing Authors

Elena Albé, MD (Chapters 5 and 6)

Waleed A. Allam, MD, PhD (Chapter 4)

David A. Goldman, MD (Chapter 9)

Anastasios John Kanellopoulos, MD (Chapter 8)

Mounir A. Khalifa, MD, PhD (Chapter 4)

Scipione Rossi, MD (Chapter 7)

William Trattler, MD (Chapter 9)

Paolo Vinciguerra, MD (Chapter 5 and 6)

R. Vinciguerra, MD (Chapters 5 and 6)

Foreword

Laser correction of refractive errors has been an evolution of science and technology that with the incorporation of complex yet rational surgical techniques, has led to today's extremely precise and sophisticated treatments. This book aims to look at the current treatment techniques of the eye's surface as used today by the top international experts in refractive surgery.

PRK has possibly evolved to a lesser degree than Lasik and the other techniques of laser vision correction, however, over the years the information on the eye's healing response, pharmacology, therapy and biomechanics have greatly improved. Many other factors have evolved as well; the clinical situation, lasers and diagnostic instruments, and surgeon experience just to name a few.

In spite of all these variables, thanks to all the new science we cover in this book, PRK now produces more stable results, with fewer complications and a better visual and functional outcome for the patient than we would have ever dreamed possible.

Lucio Buratto, MD

Introduction

Sight is a neuro-physiological process that can be broken down into two main components: the optical system of the globe and the image detection and processing of the retina and the nervous system to the occipital cortex.

Normal vision or sight is highly dependent upon the properties of the cornea—its transparency and its ability, along with the crystalline lens, to project sharp images onto the retina.

Distortion or blurring of the image may be caused by aberrations, dispersion, and/ or diffraction. Optical aberrations are the main cause of blurred vision in the human eye. Distortion induced by dispersion and diffraction are less common. In the past, optical imperfections of the eye were considered simply to be refractive errors (ie, blurred images, astigmatism, and prismatic effects that are now grouped under the heading of lower-order aberrations). Despite the fact that doctors have been aware of other aberrations, in addition to those in the lower-order category, less attention has been paid to these *higher-order aberrations.* Recently, research in the field of ophthalmology has emerged to perfect the results of refractive laser surgery to correct higher-order errors in addition to the conventional sphero-cylinder defects.

The visual benefits from attempts to correct higher-order aberrations depend on two factors. First is the importance of the limitations of human sight caused by these aberrations; the second is the precision with which these optic defects can be corrected.

A non-invasive method for evaluating the effect or visual benefit achieved by correcting the higher-order aberrations is called the adaptive optic, which we will examine in depth in Chapter 3. This device has demonstrated how the higher-order optical aberrations, in spite of the fact that they account for only approximately 10% of the total ocular optical aberrations, produce significant visual aberrations in normal eyes.[1]

This leads to the question whether an optical correction that can potentially eliminate all ocular aberrations, limiting vision visual degradation to diffraction-related blurring only, can improve perceptive vision and, if so, to what degree? The answer is subject to anatomical limits, the design of the optics, and the image detection and processing components of the human visual system.

Improvements in the optics of the eye increase the contrast and the spatial details of the retinal image. Both of these effects are pupil-dependent, the greater the diameter of the pupil, the lower the degree of contrast and the more blurred the retinal images.

The foveal area of the retina, with a diameter of approximately 0.35 mm (0.385 mm^2 or approximately 1°), contains the greatest density of cones and is the area of the retina with the highest spatial resolution (Figure 1). Moving away from the fovea, the cone density is reduced with a corresponding reduction in the spatial resolution. Thus, for the best quality, the image must be focused on the foveal area. Inside the foveal area, cones are closely packed together, and each one has a diameter of approximately 2 µm. The exact limit of maximum visual acuity is actually determined by the diameter of the fovea, the cone density, and individual biological variations. If we assume, for example, that a foveal photoreceptor has a dimension in the order of 2 to 2.5 µm (the center-center distance between two adjoining cones lies between 2 and 3 µm), and the foveal distance from the nodal point of an emmetropic eye is 16.67 mm, this receptor spatial arrangement would limit the visual acuity to between 20/10 and 20/8 (or rather 60 and 75 cycles/degree) the so-called Nyquist's Limit. The fact that the photoreceptor mosaic limits the visual acuity does not mean that objects with finer details will be invisible. Objects smaller than 20/8 can be detected by the human eye with sufficient contrast but will not be perceived in their true shape.

Given the photoreceptor's inability to recognize the details, the image will be distorted and will produce a false perception of the article (aliasing) (Figure 2). The image can assume an appearance that differs greatly from the original object itself. Therefore, a theoretical eye, without aberrations, has a visual acuity of 20/8, and a further increase in quality of the optics cannot increase visual acuity, but will only improve the contrast acuity under low lighting conditions.

These visual limitations refer to the monochromatic aberrations, given that these can be measured easily by the current diagnostic methods using an aberrometer. The limit of spatial discrimination is lower with polychromatic aberrations, due to the different wavelengths associated with a color image.

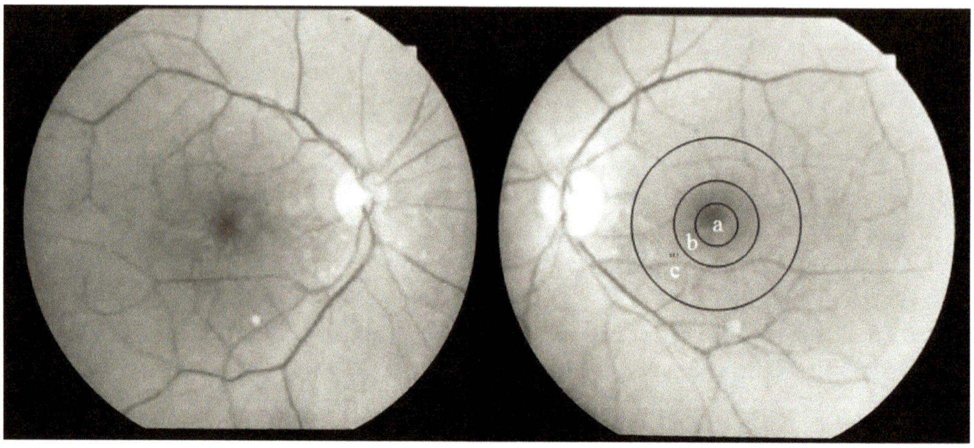

Figure 1. The macular region: (A) foveola, (B) fovea, and (C) parafoveal area.

Can the neuro-visual system benefit from any improvement to the eye's optic? There would be little gained by improving the eye's optic to limits dictated by the photoreceptor mosaic if the visual cortex is not able to perceive the improvements.

The measurement of an individual's sensitivity to distinguish grids of different spatial frequency is termed contrast sensitivity function (CSF). This CSF may be measured, under experimental conditions, with a laser fringe pattern. The reciprocal entity of the threshold is the sensitivity to contrast. The nervous system can resolve high spatial frequencies up to Nyquist's limit, with a decline in CSF at high spatial frequencies. This means that the individual needs greater contrast in order to perceive smaller details.[2-5] In an aberrated eye, a reduction in CSF equal to spatial frequency is observed. Thus, by correcting the total aberrations of the eye, it is possible to improve the spatial resolution as far as the limit permitted by the functional anatomy of the eye itself.

We wish, in our book, to present the current knowledge regarding anatomy, function, and structure of the corneal tissue as well as instruments used to measure the optical characteristics and methods of excimer laser surface refractive surgery methods and techniques.

The original goal of refractive surgery was to improve the simple focus of images on the retina. Currently, the objective is to ensure that these images are as free as possible from aberrations, even when the pupil is in mydriasis. Modification of the dioptric power of the central cornea was considered sufficient to ensure the success of the operation. Patients frequently complained, despite being corrected in sphere and cylinder with good Snellen acuity, of a loss in contrast, of appearance of halos around light sources, and of other visual disturbances that reduced the visual quality.

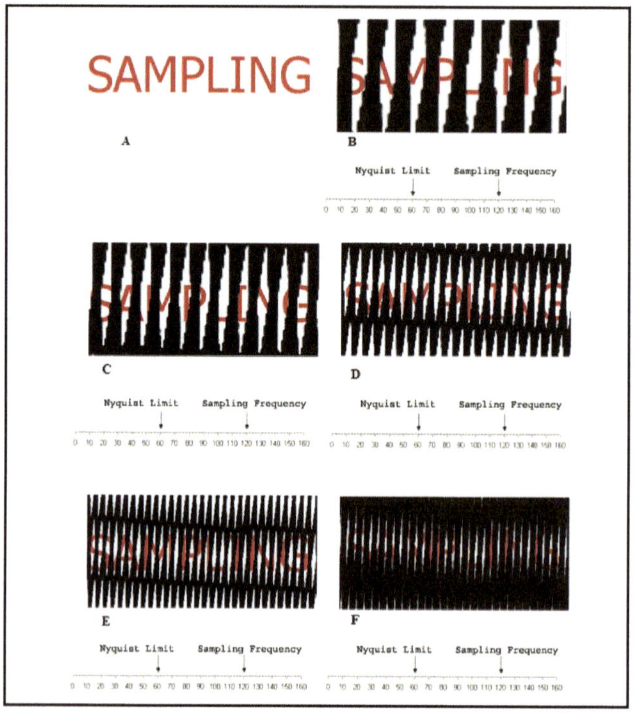

Figure 2. Retinal vision simulated by grids of 10 (A), 20 (B), 40 (C), 80 (D), and 120 (F) cycles/degrees examined by a mosaic of the foveal retinal receptors. With a spatial frequency in excess of 75 cycles/degree, the visual perception may appear distorted (aliasing), limiting the ability of the nervous system to interpret the high quality retinal image. In the example, not how it is not possible to distinguish the parallel pale and dark lines of the grid.

In clinical practice, the advent of systems to measure ocular aberrations and the increasingly detailed knowledge of the optical properties of the eye highlighted how the higher-order aberrations affect the visual performance.

Increasingly accurate ablation systems, which can reduce the induction of higher-order aberrations produced by the first systems, are now available to the refractive surgeon. Indeed, almost all of the laser systems can generate a treatment based on the ocular aberrations for a personalized treatment of the total defect.

The most advanced method for surgical correction of corneal optical aberrations is customizing the treatment based on total ocular aberrations.

It is of fundamental importance for the refractive surgeon to not only eliminate blurred vision and astigmatism but also to reduce the higher-order aberrations of the ocular optics to a minimum. Modern lasers achieve this by modifying the corneal profile and optimizing the optical quality of the surfaces. This increased ability to measure the optical and biophysical properties of the cornea along with the development of more accurate ablation systems can achieve results that stretch far beyond simply ridding the patient of glasses or contact lenses.

Part I

Chapter 1

The Corneal Surface

Lucio Buratto, MD; Stephen G. Slade, MD, FACS; Sebastiano Serrao, MD, PhD; and Marco Lombardo, MD, PhD

Anatomy

The ocular surface is the external aspect of the eye and consists of the cornea, the conjunctiva, and the lacrimal film.

The cornea is transparent, avascular, deformable, and accounts for the anterior portion of the outer layer of the eye. It is surrounded by sclera and is curved more steeply than the rest of the eye as its mean radius of curvature is less than the radius of curvature of the sclera. The cornea is the most powerful refractive element of the eye. The cornea-air interface produces the greatest modification of the refractive index of the eye. The dioptric power of the corneal surface accounts for approximately 80% of the eye's total dioptric power.

The prolate anterior surface of the cornea is in contact with the lacrimal film and the palpebral conjunctiva. Its outline is elliptical with a mean horizontal diameter of 11.7 mm (11 to 12.8 mm), 1 mm more than the vertical diameter, which has a mean value of 10.7 mm (10 to 11.5 mm). Topographically, it is possible to identify an approximately spherical central zone of 4 mm diameter, with a radius of curvature 7 to 7.5 mm and a paracentral, circular, intermediate zone, which is progressively flatter toward the limbus, approximately 2.5-mm wide. The peripheral portion, or corneal limbus, is 1 to 2 mm wide and marks the transition between the corneal and the sclero-conjunctival tissue.

The corneal epithelium consists of polystratified squamous non-keratinized epithelium, consisting of five to seven rows of cells, with a mean life cycle of 7 days; the thickness varies from 45 μm centrally to 80 μm in the periphery. Three layers can be identified: one superficial, one intermediate, and one basal. The latter rests on a thin basal membrane, Bowman's membrane, approximately 30 to 60 μm thick.

The basal layer consists of a single layer of polyhedral cells oriented with their greatest axis perpendicular to the surface (mean height: 20 μm; mean width: 10 μm). Their cytoplasm is rich with organelles, which indirectly indicates a considerable metabolic capacity. Lymphocytes, histiocytes, and Langerhans cells are visible in the basal layer.[6]

The basal cells undergo morphological and biochemical modifications as they transform into polygonal elements along with extensions and ramifications that facilitate their adhesion to each other and to the basal layers below. The intermediate layer consists of two to three rows of cells with a diameter of 25 to 30 μm and the greatest axis parallel to the corneal surface. Their cytoplasm is dense with microtubules and tono-filaments parallel to the greater cell axis. The polygonal elements are transformed into squamous cells, as they migrate toward the surface, and are

Buratto L, Slade S, Serrao S, Lombardo M. ***PRK: The Past, Present, and Future of Surface Ablation.*** *(pp. 3-10).*

organized in two to three overlying layers, parallel to the corneal surface. These form the surface of the corneal epithelium. The squamous cells are flat, with a width between 40 and 60 µm and just 4 to 6 µm thick. A key characteristic is the disintegration of the nucleus, prior to the desquamation and the low quantity of cytoplasmic organisms. They also contain a large quantity of contractile proteins, such as actin, which adhere to the plasma membrane. These cells act as a microskeleton and also facilitate cell migration.

On ultra-microscopic observation, two types of surface cells can be identified: pale cells and dark cells.[7] The dark cells are characterized by a greater number of surface microvilli than the pale cells. This can be correlated with the age of the cell. Their greater density and the length of the surface microvilli result in a greater adhesion and stability of the lacrimal film onto the epithelium surface.[8]

In spite of the fact that the corneal epithelium is subject to continual cell turnover, the process of epithelial renewal continues with no loss of contact between the layers. Lateral anchoring between cells is due to the presence of joining complexes that surround the entire cell. The basal cells are anchored by hemidesmosomes present in the basal membrane. This particular membrane is positioned immediately below the basal cells, with a non-uniform thickness of between 7 and 30 nm. The thickness of the layer tapers off toward the edge of the cornea and becomes continuous with the extremely thin basal membrane of the scleral conjunctiva.

The basal membrane is a product of extracellular secretion of the basal cells. It has the dual function of separating the epithelium from the stroma and supporting the organization of the epithelium itself. Ultra-structural observation shows that it consists of a clear anterior zone (the lamina lucida) and the posterior electron-dense zone (the lamina dense). Along with Bowman's membrane, the basal membrane forms the complex of epithelial-stromal junction.

Bowman's membrane is acellular, 8 to 14-µm thick, consisting of numerous collagen fibrils (largely type V). These are entwined and end abruptly at the limbus. Bowman's is continuous with the underlying stroma and, once it has been destroyed or photo ablated, does not regenerate.

The mechanism of adhesion of the complexes of epithelial-stromal junctions has not been completely clarified. The tonofilaments of the posterior surface of the basal cells are involved as well as other thin anchoring filaments that cut perpendicularly across the junctional complex. Analysis of these structures shows the presence of laminin, fibronectin Type IV and Type V collagen, and eparan sulfate.

The corneal stroma, which represents 90% of the entire corneal thickness, consists primarily of a foundation substance containing the cells of the parenchyma, the keratocytes, and the collagen lamellas.

The foundation substance, secreted by the keratocytes, consists of proteoglycans, glycoproteins, other soluble proteins, water, and mineral salts. The proteoglycans and the glycoproteins have an axial position with respect to the collagen fibrils and surround them like a sheath.[9] Keratin sulfate and dermatan sulfate are the main constituents of the stroma's foundation substance.

Each of the collagen lamellas is approximately 2-µm thick. There are approximately 300 lamellae in the central corneal sections and approximately 500 in the peripheral sections. Each lamella is a lateral arrangement of several collagen fibrils (mean thickness 31 nm under the electronic microscope and 81 nm under the atomic force microscope).[7,10] The most common collagen fibrils in the corneal stroma are called Type I (68% of the stroma's dry weight).

Type III, V, VI, XII, and XVI collagen fibers have also been isolated. The lamellae are formed by neatly organized individual bundles of fibrils of mean thickness 81 nm ± 20 nm (range: 48 to 113 nm), axial D-periodicity of 67 nm ± 10 nm observed under the atomic force microscope (Figure 1-1),[11] and 10 to 250 nm observed under the electronic microscope (D-periodicity of 60 to 70 nm).

Inside the bundles, the individual fibers run parallel to each other. Collagen fibers of thickness 2 to 5 µm and an axial D-periodicity superior to 68 nm have also been observed and are called fibrous long spacing collagen.

Collagen fibrils possess a high refractive index and are believed to actually diffract light. The transparency of the corneal tissue can therefore be attributed to the ultrastructural order of the small even diameter of the collagen fibers and the uniformity of the bundling.[7,12-14] The orientation of the collagen fibrils in a normal cornea is extremely complex. For the most part, at the limbus, the fibrils are arranged in a circle, tangential to the limbus itself.

The thickness of this limbal ring is greater in the lower region and smaller in the upper regions. In the stroma, the preferential infero-superior and naso-longitudinal orientation of the vertical and horizontal collagen arches can be observed.[14] This orientation is more uniform in the posterior stroma compared to the anterior stroma. In contrast, the anterior stroma

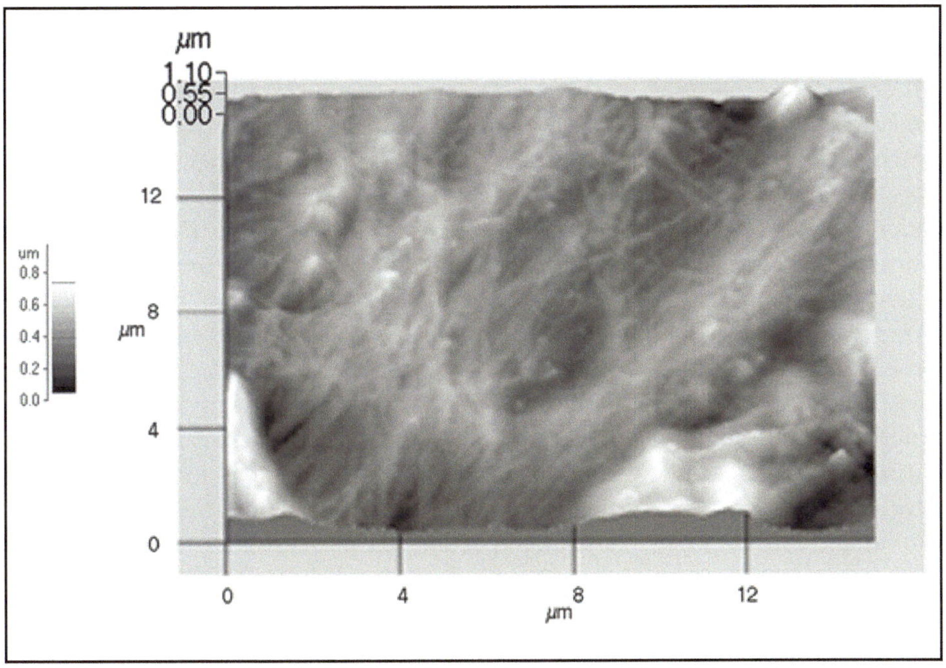

Figure 1-1. At high magnification, the AFM three-dimensional representation provides a high-quality topographical map of the anterior stromal features. The organization of the collagen fibrils in bundles and their parallel arrangement may be observed between the granular structures. Scale image: 15 x 15 µm.

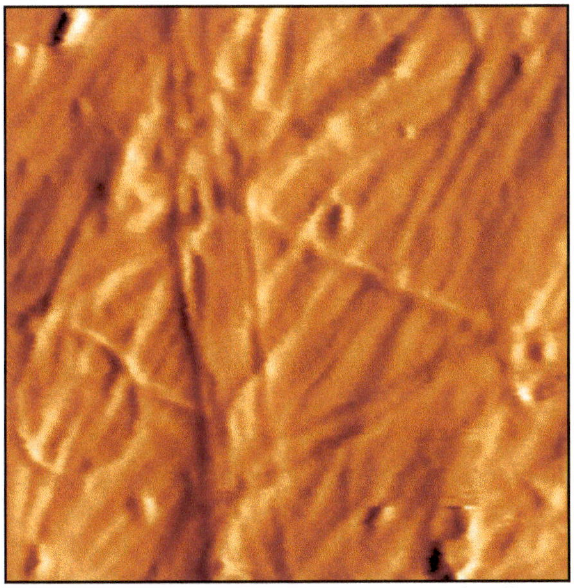

Figure 1-2. AFM image of human corneal collagen fibers, isolated mechanically (in Triton X-100) and deposited on mica.

appears to be more rigid than the posterior stroma with closer, tighter bonds between the collagen lamellae (Figure 1-2).[15]

The keratocytes lie between the collagen lamellae. These cells ensure continuous synthesis of the collagen fibrils and the extracellular matrix. The cells are flat and star-shaped with a diameter of approximately 109 nm. Their numerous cytoplasmic extensions connect and join with the adjacent cells. The keratocytes probably communicate through gap junctions, producing functional synchrony.[16] Keratocytes are cells that differentiate and proliferate under certain environmental conditions. They play a role of primary importance in the scarring processes of the corneal surfaces, following any type of corneal surgery.

The cornea also contains a dense network of two types of sensory nerve fibers, which originate from the ophthalmic branch of the trigeminal nerve (fifth cranial nerve). The bodies of these cells are located in the upper cervical ganglion. Quantitatively, these nerve fibers are more numerous than the sympathetic nerve fibers. The naso-ciliary nerve, a branch of the ophthalmic nerve, penetrates the orbit through the superior orbital fissure. It splits into at least two branches prior to cutting through the sclera and subsequently runs parallel to the scleral plane. As they pass through the eye, the nerves branch again and eventually reach the supra-choroidal space, where they form a dense network. At the limbus, the nerves entwine with the sympathetic nerve fibers. Finally, inside the cornea, the nerve fibers, which are located for the most part in the middle section of the stroma, proceed forward to form a dense sub-epithelial plexus. They then cross Bowman's membrane and, as free nerve endings, reach the layers of the corneal epithelium. The nerve endings have a plexiform distribution, with greater density in the central cornea with respect to the peripheral areas. The fibers are not coated in a myelin sheath, and the intra-epithelial fibers also lack the Schwann's sheath. In the stroma, the nerve fibers are organized into bundles that lie parallel to the collagen lamellae. In the epithelium, the fibers create a fine network, which surrounds the cells in the basal and intermediate layers. No nerves run through the deep layers of the corneal parenchyma.

The stromal-corneal nerve system can be examined in vivo at the slit lamp. Its function can be investigated using an extensiometer. Confocal microscopy of the cornea is currently the best option for fine analysis of the stromal and sub-epithelial nerve cells.

The nerve system of the cornea is considered to be vital for maintaining the structure and the function of corneal tissue. It has been suggested that the nerve endings operate by secreting neuro-peptides. Studies have shown that synaptic nerve endings in rats will stimulate epithelial proliferation under normal physiological conditions and following traumatic injury. Numerous experimental studies have demonstrated how sensory denervation modifies the re-epithelialization process.[17]

The lacrimal film is a thin layer of liquid that covers the corneal and conjunctival epithelium. It is 4 to 7 µm thick and is slightly alkaline and hypotonic with respect to plasma. The tear film consists of three separate layers: the most superficial lipid layer, which is approximately 0.1 µm thick; the intermediate aqueous layer, which forms the most conspicuous component of the lacrimal liquid, approximately 4 to 7 µm thick; and the mucous layer, which is closely correlated to the glycocalyx of the cells on the cornea's surface, approximately 0.02 to 0.05 µm thick.

The lipids in the lacrimal film are secreted by glands in the eyelids: the meibomian, Zeiss, and Moll. The lipid film consists of two layers: one is polar and more superficial; the other nonpolar layer is in contact with the aqueous layer below. The lacrimal lipids contain esters of cholesterol, wax esters, phospholipids, and triglycerides and free fatty acids. The lipid layer tends to delay evaporation and reduces the surface tension of the lacrimal film. It also plays an important role in maintaining an adequate thickness of the lacrimal film itself. The aqueous layer controls the oxygenation of the corneal surface. When the eyes are open, the oxygen dissolved in the lacrimal film has the same partial atmospheric pressure. The aqueous layer also contains metabolites necessary for the fermentation processes of the cell epithelium, immunoglobulins, and antibacterial enzymes. The mucous layer consists of mucin processed by the goblet cells in the conjunctiva, the mucous crypts of Henle, and the Manz glands. It has been suggested that the mucous component secreted by the conjunctiva forms an intermediate layer between the aqueous component of the lacrimal film and the glycocalyx of the corneal cells. This reduces the surface tension in the internal layer of lacrimal liquid and produces maximum humidification of the corneal epithelium.

The surface of the pre-corneal lacrimal film is the first and outermost ocular surface. Combined with a uniform corneal lacrimal film, it forms a single integrated optic complex with a single refractive index. A number of clinical studies have attempted to correlate the rheological characteristics of the lacrimal film to visual performance, demonstrating how a non-uniform lacrimal film, reduced lacrimal thickness, and sporadic blinking are correlated to an increase in higher-order aberrations (Figure 1-3).[18,19] These are also an important source of error in the measurements of ocular aberration and aberrations of the first outermost corneal surface.

Epithelial Renewal

The corneal epithelium is constantly renewed. This integrated, complex balance between cell proliferation, migration, and death supports the transparency and the optic properties of the corneal surface. The process of epithelial renewal is based on four essential phases: cell division, cell migration, cell adhesion to the basal membrane, and stromal-epithelial interaction.

Cell division occurs in the basal cell layer. The gradual upward and outward movement of the new cells that reach the surface culminates in the desquamation or shedding of the old cells from the surface.

In the past, it was not clear how the mitotic activity of the basal layer cells managed to maintain a fully coated surface of epithelial cells. Thanks to studies by Davanger and Evenson,[20] the parent cell of the corneal epithelium was identified in the limbus. This ring-shaped peripheral region is approximately 1 to 2-mm wide and marks the boundary between clear cornea and bulbar conjunctiva. It also contains the deep Vogt epithelial grooves that penetrate the highly vascularized papillary stroma.

The parent cells are a stable population of undifferentiated cells (pluripotent stem cells) that undergo the standard "asymmetrical" cell division, giving rise to two populations of daughter cells. One of these populations will continue to maintain the stem cell pool; the second will differentiate into cells called "transitory amplifier cells." These, in turn, will divide

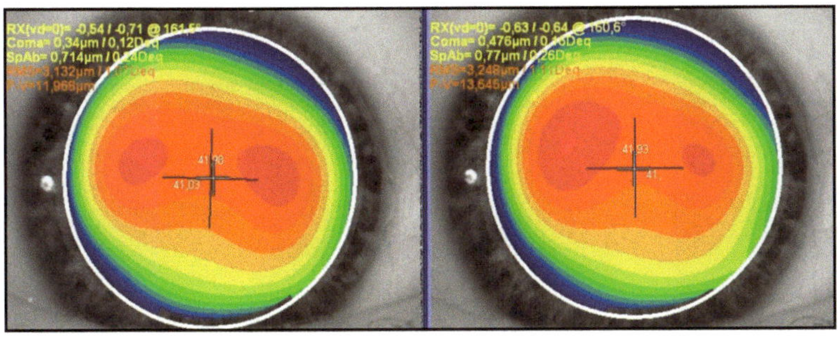

Figure 1-3. Corneal aberrometric map between two successive blinks. Note the modification in the structure of the optic aberrations, with a considerable increase in the high order aberrations, coma in particular. A repeated and accurate aquisition of the aberrometric map is the first step to precise knowledge regarding the error in the patient's wavefront.

several times prior to the final differentiation into basal epithelial cells.[21] Schofield first proposed the idea of a "stem cell niche."[22] Schofield suggested that the cell pool is housed under conditions that will prevent the differentiation. Numerous experimental studies have highlighted how cell differentiation is closely associated with apoptosis or programmed cell death. The fibroblasts in the stroma of the corneal limbus are different from those of the central cornea and are able to secrete anti-apoptopic factors.[23] As confirmation of this hypothesis, numerous autocrine and aparacribe complexes have been observed; they are mediated by cytokine and operate between the epithelial cells and the stromal cells of the limbus and the central cornea.[24]

Thoft and Friend[25] suggested the "X, Y, Z hypothesis" for epithelial renewal. "X" represents the proliferation of the epithelial basal cells, "Y" is the centripetal migration of the cells, and "Z" is the desquamation of the surface cells. In this model, the desquamated cells are replaced by the limbal stem cells through mitotic activity. The loss of the surface cells by desquamation has been estimated as 5 to 15 cells per minute for the entire corneal surface.[26]

The process of epithelial cell renewal is influenced by numerous factors including xerophthalmia,[27] corneal denervation, inflammation, the use of contact lenses,[28] and the presence of growth factors. A model designed to provide an accurate description of the epithelial regeneration process must consider the density of the proliferative cells of the basal layer, the density of the surface quiescent cells of the surface layers, and the concentration of metabolites that regulate cell proliferation and migration.[29] Thus, any epithelial abrasion or any wounds to the corneal surface without involvement of Bowman's membrane and the stroma below will heal symmetrically.[30]

The normal process of re-epithelialization can be split into two phases: a latent phase and a linear phase. The latent phase lasts approximately 5 hours during which the advance of the re-epithelialization front is minimal. During the linear phase, there is a linear, symmetrical progression of the re-epithelialization front on the entire corneal surface. During the initial phase, the depth of the epithelial front is reduced to a single layer of cells, demonstrating that cell loss through desquamation is greater than cell regeneration. During this initial period, epithelial cover occurs through the lateral displacement of the cells into the surrounding areas. During the second phase, the mean speed of cell migration is constant and independent of the shape and the dimensions of the epithelial abrasion, suggesting that cell movement is the limiting factor in this phase, characterized by mitosis of the basal cells.[31]

Locally secreted growth factors regulate and integrate the complex mechanism of re-epithelialization with systemic, hormonal, and neurogenic influences. The mitotic activity of the corneal epithelium follows a circadian cycle with peaks shown in rats at approximately 9 am and at 1 pm.[32] Estil and colleagues[33] demonstrated that epithelial regeneration was faster in rat eyes when the other eye had been damaged or scratched 1 week earlier. In patients who have undergone photorefractive keratectomy (PRK), re-epithelialization was faster in the second eye when operated 1 week after the first.[34] New information regarding the kinetics associated with re-epithelialization has come to light in recent years, thanks to the use of electronic microscopic and immunohistological techniques that highlight the numerous ultrastructural factors involved in the process. Epithelial regeneration is a primary source of anchoring molecules and formation of the basal membrane that is organized once the epithelium has assumed its normal multistratified architecture.[35] "Joining complexes," between cells, support the epithelium. These renewed cells can immediately form appropriate connections with the adjoining cells, with no reduction in the permeability of the corneal surface to external agents.[36]

Numerous clinical and experimental studies, performed on intact corneas subjected to photorefractive surgery, have demonstrated how the degree of smoothness of the surface is the most important

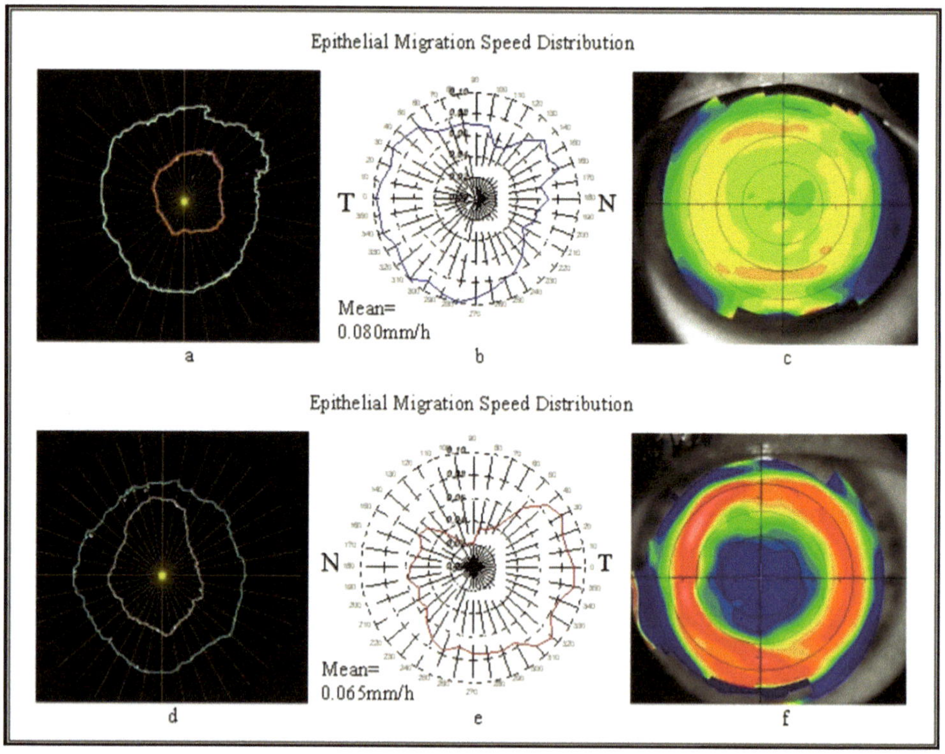

Figure 1-4. (A) and (D) are the re-epithelialization fronts 20 and 40 hours after surgery. (B) and (E) describe the distribution of the radial velocity of the corneal epithelium along 36 meridians. (C) and (F) represent the tangential maps one month from surgery.

variable in correct epithelial healing. The uniformity of the first outermost corneal surface (Figure 1-4) and the postoperative visual result are correlated to the regeneration of the epithelium. This phenomenon is associated with the reduction in the activation of the cascade of events associated with the epithelial-stromal remodeling.

Epithelial-Stromal Remodeling of Surfaces Ablated With the Excimer Laser

The variability of the results of surface corneal refractive surgery with excimer lasers can be attributed to the response of the corneal tissue to the surgical procedure.

Numerous factors, correlated to the surgical technique and to the biophysical response of the cornea, can influence the remodeling mechanism of the ablated corneal surface. Techniques and physical properties associated with the laser that may influence the remodeling mechanisms include the humidity and temperature of the operating room,[37] the technique used to remove the epithelium prior to the ablation,[38] the uniformity and profile of the laser beam,[39] the pulse frequency[40] and the beam fluence,[41] the diameter of the spot,[42] molecular debris deposited on the stromal surface following every pulse of the laser beam hitting the corneal surface, whether VES is applied during surgery (smoothing),[43,44] the angle of the corneal plane with respect to the angle of incidence of the laser pulses, and eye movements. All of these factors can influence the final result of the ablated surfaces, which may not be perfectly smooth, a major factor in the epithelium and stromal healing process. Rapid epithelial healing is the most important and essential condition for excellent epithelial-stromal scarring.[45]

Numerous experimental studies examined the factors involved in the individual biophysical response process following treatment with the excimer laser. These include cytokines such as tumor necrosis factor α and β (TNF-α and TNF-β), the transforming growth factor β (TGF-β), epidermal growth factor (EGF),[46] the platelet-activating factor (PAF),[47] and the fibroblast growth factor (FGF), proteolytic enzymes such as metalloproteases, variations in the components of the extracellular matrix, and the apoptosis mechanism.

Apoptosis of the keratocytes lying below the ablated stromal surface is the earliest phase observed in the cascade of events in the epithelial-stromal remodeling process.[48] Every alteration to the apoptosis process can have a negative influence on the remodeling process of the ablated corneal surfaces. There is a reduction in the keratocyte population of the anterior stroma, immediately following stromal ablation that is mediated by apoptosis. Numerous experimental studies have identified the source of cytokines responsible for the activation of this process in the damaged epithelium. The process is observed in every traumatic event and infection of the corneal surface. It is probably a nonspecific defense mechanism in response to every type of injury or damage to the corneal surface. Leukocytes have been observed on the ablated stromal surface 12 hours after corneal abrasions. These cells have been observed in the deeper layers after 24 hours.[49] Through paracrine signals, the leukocytes can activate the migration of the epithelial cells and activate the keratocytes. Between 12 and 24 hours from the traumatic event, the keratocytes surrounding the injured area will differentiate and proliferate, secreting the components of the fundamental matrix and regulating the stratification of the overlying epithelium.

New synthesis of stroma, following photo-ablation, is mediated by keratocyte activity and is the biological key to refractive stability following each treatment. Refractive regression is always correlated with an increase in the stromal thickness. To date, no clinical studies have demonstrated an association between an increase in epithelial thickening and regression.[50] The development of corneal haze[51] is not correlated with the process of regression, suggesting that the two phenomena depend on two different biological mechanisms. Studies performed with confocal microscopy show that haze would appear to be correlated to the density and the cellular volume of keratocytes in the anterior stroma, as though the modification in transparency of the photo-ablated stroma largely depends on an intracellular component, rather than deposits of an abnormal extracellular component.[52] Under electronic microscopy, in addition to the increased density of the keratocytes, the lateral arrangement of the collagen fibrils in the anterior stroma appears to be completely irregular[53] in the first postsurgery months. At the end of the first month postsurgery, the morphology of the keratocytes in the anterior stroma closely resembles myofibroblasts.

Numerous in vitro studies have investigated the relationship between the activated keratocytes and the corneal epithelium. The primary activation of the keratocytes of the anterior stroma (into fibroblasts) is initiated by a lack of contact with the epithelium above. The successive stratification of the epithelium is accompanied by the differentiation of the fibroblasts into myofibroblasts with contractile properties, suggesting that the activity of this differentiated cellular phenotype drives the production of paracrine-type cell signals that modulate the epithelium.[54] Six months after surgery, the cell density and morphology are similar to that of a normal population of keratocytes.[55]

The regulation of keratocyte apoptosis is currently the subject of numerous clinical and experimental research trials. The idea is exciting; inhibiting or reducing the initial apoptosis may attenuate the phenomenon of epithelial-stromal re-modeling, improving the accuracy of every operation of corneal refractive surgery. The result might be improved by applying molecules to the corneal surface to inhibit the apoptosis mechanisms or to indirectly regulate the cell response through an improvement to the ablated profile and a more homogeneous distribution of the laser's energy on the stromal surface. Optimizing the complex process of the epithelial and stromal remodeling would require a thorough knowledge of the numerous variables involved in the phenomenon.[56]

There are two main research objectives: first, the rapid closure of the epithelium and, second, the regulation of the keratocyte activation. For the latter, much greater knowledge of molecular biology is essential. Rapid epithelial progression on the stromal bed is possible when new techniques are used. This is termed *advanced surface ablation* (ASA) and includes smoothing and/or wavefront-guided ablations and will be examined more closely in Chapter 3. A smoother ablated stromal surface forms the basis for a better refractive and visual result. It leads to greater predictability and stability of the surgical result and better visual performance. The reason for the more accurate result is the rapid progression of the re-epithelialization and an earlier closure of the epithelium and the successive reduction in the phenomena of epithelial stromal remodeling.[57]

A smooth surface following ablation is the primary objective to prevent abnormal remodeling of the epithelium and stroma that may result in an increase in higher-order aberrations. Uniform distribution of the intensity of the laser energy over the entire treatment zone is the first and essential condition for achieving a smooth surface.

From the first article produced by Trokel and colleagues, published in 1983,[58] numerous studies have defined the efficacy and the safety levels associated with laser treatments and the ultramicroscopic

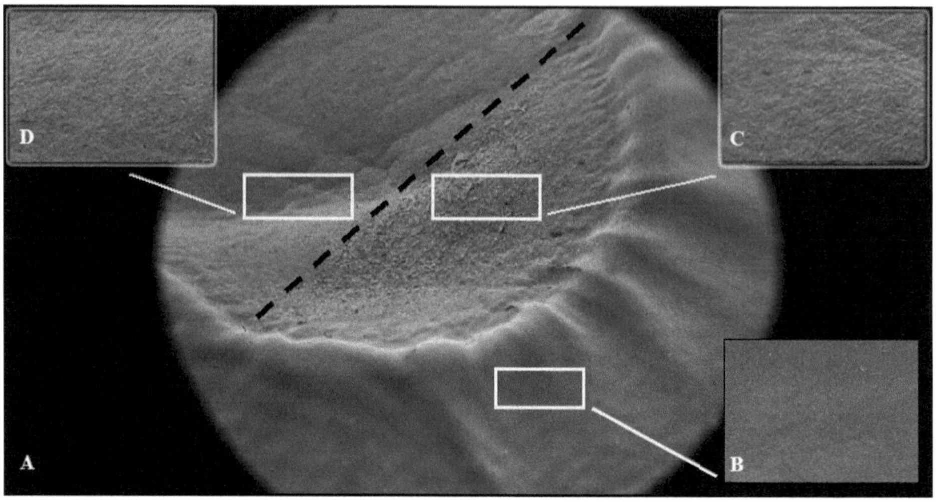

Figure 1-5. (A) Scanning electron microscope image (magnification 20x) of a pig cornea ablated with an excimer laser. (B) The corneal epithelium (250x). (C) Magnification of the area ablated with the standard technique (250x). (D) Half of the corneal plane subjected to smoothing immediately following the standard ablation.

characteristics of the ablated surfaces.[59-62] Images of the anterior stroma from the atomic force microscope or from the electronic microscope, acquired following ablation, showed micro-irregularities of the treated surfaces (Figure 1-5). The post-laser topographical modifications can be directly connected to the impact the laser beam has on the surfaces.[63,64] The micro-granular structures are assumed to be postablative debris and ruptured fibers. Some authors have suggested fragments of matter are introduced when aqueous boils during ablation. These are associated with the thermal effects of the laser.

Chapter 2

Optical and Mechanical Properties of the Cornea

Lucio Buratto, MD; Stephen G. Slade, MD, FACS; Sebastiano Serrao, MD, PhD; and Marco Lombardo, MD, PhD

Optical Aberrations

Optical aberration is the term used to describe every distortion and deviation of the retinal image induced by the surfaces of the ocular system. In a perfect eye, every infinitesimal point in the surrounding environment must correspond to a point on the retina. In actual fact, the perfect eye does not exist, and perfect vision is an impossible objective. The best possible result in the visualization of the outside world is limited by diffraction. The diffracted light wave converges onto a small finite spot called the airy disk. Generally speaking, each eye perceives greater distortion from diffraction due to the aberrations affecting its optical surfaces. Current research in visual optics is changing our outlook considerably and is modifying how we perceive the eye's optical system. In the past, the imperfections of the eye's optical system were simply considered to be errors of the refraction: myopia, hyperopia, astigmatism, and prismatic effects. At the time of writing, the ocular optical imperfections have been re-examined against the theory of wavefront light propagation. They are now described and classed as lower- or higher-order optical aberrations. Lower-order aberrations include refractive defects that can be corrected with spectacles or standard contact lenses, while higher-order aberrations include spherical aberrations, coma, and all aberrations that are classed under the heading of irregular astigmatism or defects that cannot be corrected with commercially available spectacles or lenses.

Optical aberrations can be split further into monochromatic or polychromatic. Monochromatic aberrations are associated with a specific wavelength, while polychromatic refers to aberrations of a light beam as it passes through the ocular dioptric surfaces. Polychromatic aberration is caused by the dispersion of light in the various media it crosses: the cornea, the aqueous, the crystalline lens, and the vitreous. Dispersion is simply a variation in the refractive index of a substance in relation to the wavelength of the light crossing it. White light will be split into the various colors of the visible spectrum.

Understanding optical aberrations requires knowledge of the physics behind the phenomena and the instruments developed to express it. First, it is essential to understand the wavefront concept. Light consists of moving electromagnetic waves, and the wavefront is a continuous surface that propagates perpendicular to the direction of the light rays (Figure 2-1). Ocular optical aberrations are normally expressed as an error of the wavefront as it enters the pupil. They are defined as the modification of the light beam that passes through the optical media of the eye under examination. In the event the wavefront is a plane connecting all the points

Buratto L, Slade S, Serrao S, Lombardo M. *PRK: The Past, Present, and Future of Surface Ablation.* (pp. 11-24).

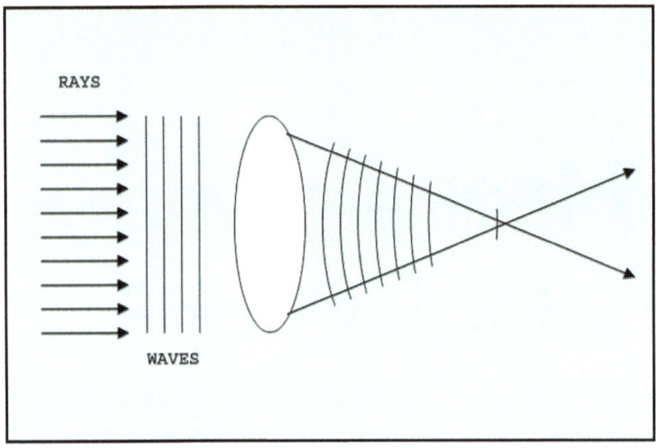

Figure 2-1. According to the wavefront theory, the light propagates in the atmosphere perpendicular to the direction of the rays. The wavefront is a surface and not a line.

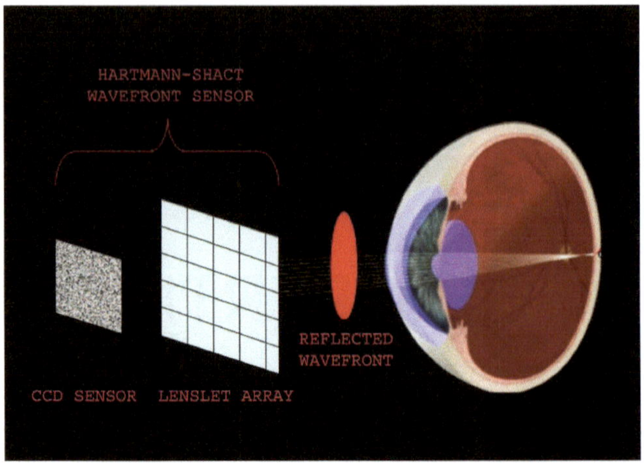

Figure 2-2. The aberrometer constructed according to the Hartmann-Shack principle exploits a grid of micro-lenses to reconstruct the wavefront of the eye under examination. A video sensor (CCD) captures an image of the collated dots for computer analysis.

of a light wave propagated in the same phase, the aberration of the wavefront is defined as a deviation of the wavefront for the reference surface. The eye's reference surface is defined as the curved surface closest to the wavefront. It originates at the tip of the Gaussian image where light passing through the eye would be perfectly in focus. In the human eye, the curved reference surface is a sphere, with the center of curvature located on the external segment of the photoreceptors. The distance between the ideal wavefront and that reflected by the eye under examination is the error of the wavefront and is quantified with the expression W(x,y) that expresses the error of the wavefront defined by the coordinates (x,y) above the pupil.

In a clinical situation, ocular optical aberrations are measured with instruments called *aberrometers*. There are numerous techniques used to measure the corneal and ocular aberrations. Consequently, there are various classifications relative to the aberrometers in the clinical environment. Wavefront sensors are split into subjective and objective, or alternately on the basis of the optical information measured. The latest classification of aberrometers refers to the ocular optical structure involved in the measurements, and, consequently, we can identify ocular aberrometers and aberrometers for the corneal first surfaces. The subjective analyzers require a response from the patient, which may prove to be a limiting factor. Objective sensors exploit imaging systems that analyze the optical information relayed from the eye under examination.

The Shack-Hartmann aberrometer (an objective sensor) is the most popular instrument used in clinical practice. This machine illuminates the foveal area with a low-energy laser light source to produce a map of the wavefront reflected by the foveal area. The result is defined by the deviation of the rays with respect to their ideal position and is not distorted by ocular optics as summarized in Figure 2-2.

The aberrometric systems available today exploit "a criterion of simplicity"; they analyze the differences between the wavefront measured and the ideal wavefront, a value referred to as the "wavefront error." One useful interpretation of aberration maps refers to the errors in the optical path length (OPL). OPL is a measurement of the number of oscillations of a light wave that propagates from point A to point B. This is an important concept as light rays emitted from a source propagate in many different directions; however, if all of the light rays have the same OPL, every ray will have the same number of oscillations. As a result, the light at the extremity of every ray will have the same temporal phase, and this group of points with a common phase represents a wavefront of light. A propagating wavefront of light is defined by a collection of points in space that are found at the same OPL of a common light source. To define the aberration of an optical system, the OPL of a ray that passes through any point (x,y) of the pupil plane can be compared to a main ray, which passes through the center of the pupil (0,0) as this light ray is not deviated nor distorted along its path. The result is the OPD (Figure 2-3). In a perfect optical system, the OPL will be the same for all light rays that travel from a point on an object to a point on the image; so the OPD is 0 for all positions (x,y) on the pupil. These rays will have the same phase and will therefore aggregate constructively to produce the perfect image. For an eye focused on infinity, the ideal

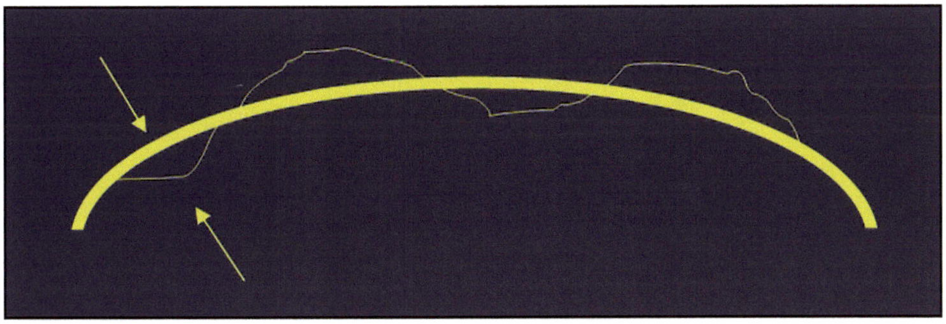

Figure 2-3. Illustration of the meaning of the wavefront. The continuous curve represents the reference wavefront. The curved dotted line, the wavefront under examination. The difference between the two wavefronts is the wavefront error or the optical path difference (OPD).

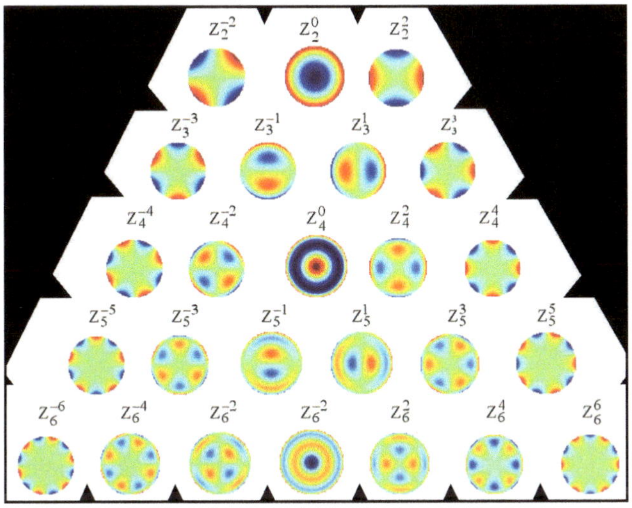

Figure 2-4. Indices for Zernike's modes used to systematically represent the structure of the eye's aberration.

wavefront exiting from an aberration-free eye is flat and circular.

On the other hand, light that passes through different points on the pupil will arrive at the destination in different phases. Consequently, the system is aberrated, and the quality of the image will be distorted. So, if we consider aberrations as being the differences in OPL, it stands to reason that the aberrations could derive from qualitative and quantitative anomalies of the lacrimal film, the cornea, the aqueous humor, the crystalline lens, the vitreous body, de-centering or inclination of the various optical components of the eye, and each component's relationship to the others. OPD is therefore a measurement that is correlated to W(x,y) and, consequently,

$$W(x,y) = -OPD(x,y)$$

A map of OPD, which crosses the pupil plane, is therefore equivalent to the mathematical expression W (x,y) where x and y are the horizontal and vertical axes relative to the shape of the aberrated wavefront that exits from the eye. The value W(x,y) is normally measured in microns.[65,66]

A mathematical method for classifying the maps of ocular (or corneal) aberrations considers every map as the adjusted sum of the fundamental shapes or the basic functions. Zernike polynomials are the ideal tool for describing the shape of the wavefront affected by optical aberrations that pass through the pupil and that are circular in shape. These groups of mathematical expressions are the product of two functions—one of which depends solely on the ρ radius of a point on the pupil, and the other depends solely on the θ meridian of a point on the pupil plane. The first function is a simple polynomial of the nth degree, and the second is the harmonic of a sine or cosine. The *dual index model* Z_n^m is useful to describe these functions accurately; the index *"n"* describes the higher power (order) of the radial polynomials and the index "m," which describes the Azimuthal frequency of the sinusoidal component.

The basic Zernike functions, or modes or terms, are systematically grouped on a pyramid-shaped periodic table (Figure 2-4). Each line of the pyramid corresponds to a given order of the polynomial of the function, and each column corresponds to the different Azimuthal frequency. By convention, the harmonics in the cosine phase are identified with a "plus" sign while those in the sine phase are identified with a "minus" sign. The unit of measurement for every Zernike coefficient is the micron, occasionally referred to as "λ," and refers to wavelength. The basic Zernike functions refer to a system of Cartesian axes. Typically, the system of reference coordinates is oriented to the right, and for the eye, the coordinates originate at the center of the pupil. The bilateral symmetry of the structure of the eye's aberrations should produce W(x,y) for the left eye equivalent to W(-x,y) for the right eye. If W is expressed as a series of Zernike functions, then the bilateral symmetry will produce Zernike coefficients of different signs for the two eyes for all the modes with uneven symmetry with respect to the y-axis.

The advantage of this description of the ocular aberrometric map is that immediate visualization of the relative adjustment is possible for each of the

Figure 2-5. Representation of a high contrast logMAR ottotype with the Zernike modes. Each Zernike term is aberrated by 0.25 μm of RMS wavefront error. The last line of the ottotype indicates 20/20 (logMAR 0.0).

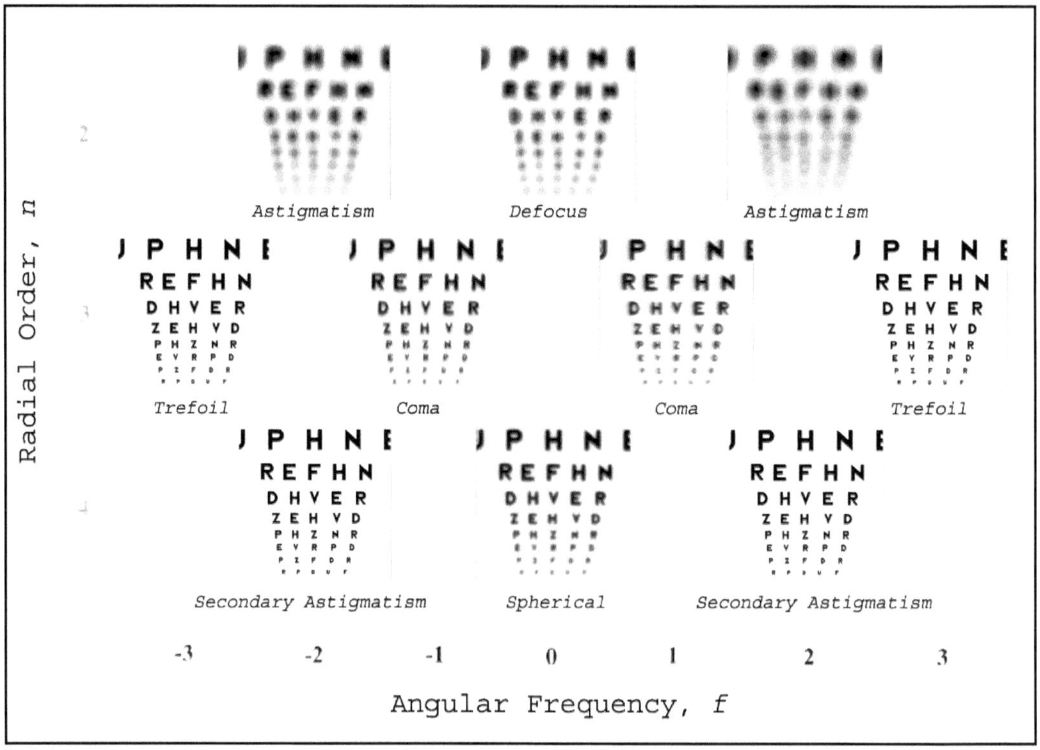

Zernike functions that will compete to form the aberrative structure of the eye. The lowest order of Zernike polynomials is familiar quantities: Z_0 is a flat piston; Z_1^1 and Z_1^{-1} represent an inclination along the vertical and horizontal axes (Prisma). Z_2^0 represents the blurring or the spherical refractive error (the common "refractive defect" referred to in the classical texts of optical physiopathology); Z_2^2 and Z_2^{-2} represent the astigmatism—orthogonal (with- or against-the-rule) and oblique (45/135 gradi). The superior orders, from the third upward, are classified as higher-order aberrations. With the assistance of the Zernike decomposition, it is possible to identify the relative influence that each optical aberration has on vision, or, rather, it is possible to quantify the degree to which a single aberrometric defect can distort the retinal image. By observing the value of the coefficients, it is possible to identify which aberrations have a greater influence on the total error of the wavefront in the specific eye. The influence of the different coefficients in reducing the quality of the retinal image is well known. Using adaptive optics visual simulators, for a specific fixed value of RMS, the different impact of each coefficient of Zernike on vision can be visualized.[67] If the lower-order (sphero-cylindrical defect) aberrations are excluded, the third- and fourth-order Zernike coefficients will have a greater negative effect on vision quality with respect to all of the other higher-order aberrations (Figure 2-5). Studies performed on populations of emmetropic or emmetropized patients demonstrated that 91% of the ocular optical aberrations lie within the first two Zernike orders, and 99% within the first four orders. The correction of the first 14 Zernike functions would, therefore, be sufficient to reduce visual blurring tending toward diffraction (Figure 2-6).[68,69]

It is also well-known that the value of the ocular optical aberrations varies over time. If we exclude intrinsic errors associated with the instrumental measurements, the degree of the variability can be observed in the properties of the ocular optical surfaces, the lacrimal film, the corneal surface, the pupil, the crystalline lens, and the vitreous body. The variability also depends on the specific Zernike order and the time factor.[70] Over minutes and hours, the variability of the higher-order coefficients is minimal. Even in the long-term (over months), there is no significant variation in RMS (±0.08 μm). It has also been observed that for a given accommodative state, the aberration of the wavefront is essentially stable. As the patient ages, on the other hand, there is a predictable increase in ocular aberrations. A number of studies have shown how the total variance of the aberrations of third and fourth order increases with age, even if the increase is relatively small, particularly when compared to aberrations induced by every type of corneal incision. Senile modifications to the cornea and the crystalline lens are responsible for deterioration in the quality of the images (Figure 2-7).[71]

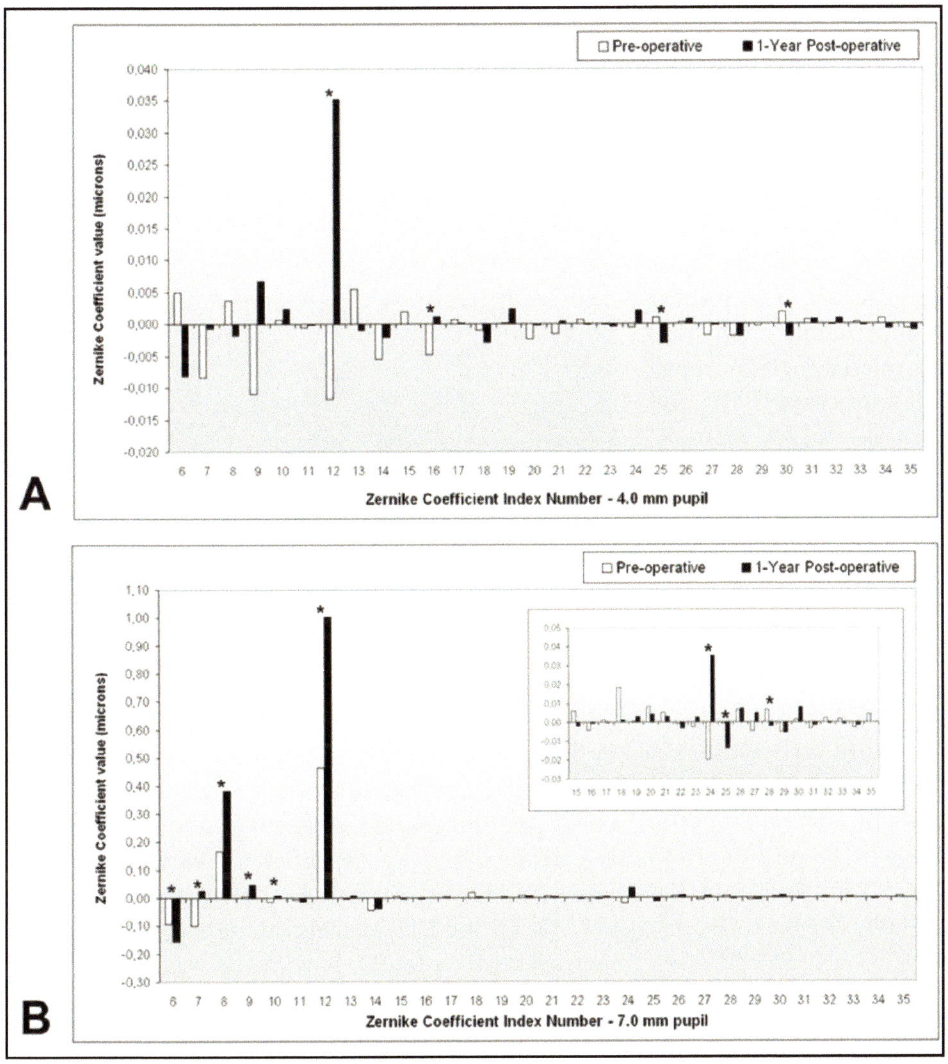

Figure 2-6. Zernike coefficients up to the 7th order in a population of 30 myopic eyes, before and a year after photorefractive keratectomy for a pupil of 4 mm (A) and 7 mm (B). The coefficients with uneven asymmetry around the y-axis have their sign (+ or -) inverted for right eyes prior to calculating the average result. The greater influence of the ocular wavefront error is limited, both before and after surgery, with the first 4 of the Zernike orders.

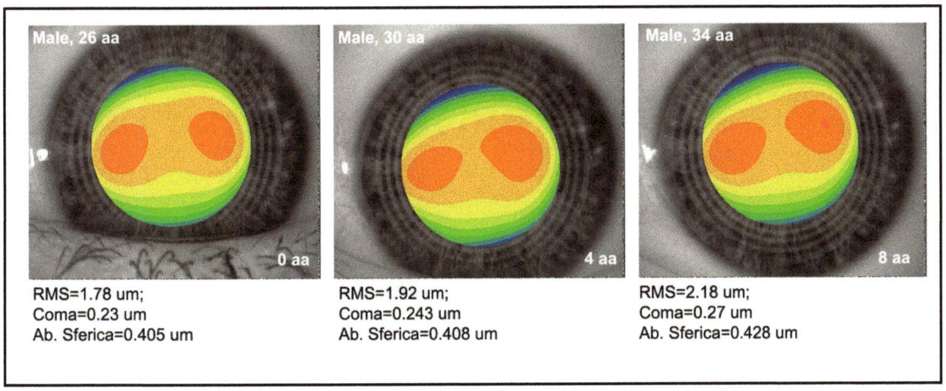

Figure 2-7. Example of the total aberration of the corneal wavefront in the eye of a young adult over a 9-year period (pupil of 7.0 mm).

The rapid fluctuations in the aberration of the wavefront (in seconds or minutes) can be correlated to the stability of the lacrimal film and accommodation.

In addition to the description of the ocular optical properties using Zernike polynomials, there are other objective methods that can describe ocular optical quality. These measurement methods have been developed to compensate for some of the disadvantages associated with the Zernike polynomials used to represent ocular wavefront error. As mentioned above, Zernike coefficients can reveal the influence that each optical aberration has on the total wavefront error. However, they do not reveal specific optical aberration impact on visual function. Moreover, if we consider eyes with numerous higher-order optical aberrations, for example, patients affected by keratoconus or following perforating keratoplasty, the accuracy of Zernike expansion will be considerably less.

New objective methods for measuring optical quality can be split into indices that describe the eye's optical properties (indices for the pupillary plane) and indices that describe the effects these properties have on the image quality. The indices for the image plane can be split further into maps of the quality of the image in reference to an object point, for example, point spread function (PSF), and the index of image quality on the grid, for example, optical transfer function (OTF). In optics, the PSF describes the effect of the optical aberrations in relation to the dominion of space. OTF describes these effects in the dominion of frequencies.[72] The main difference between the indices for the pupillary plane and the indices for the image plane is that the former describe the error of the ocular wavefront on the pupillary plane and the latter describe it on the retinal plane. The most well-known index for the pupil plane is the root-mean-square (RMS) of the wavefront error calculated for the entire pupil, RMSw. RMSw is the standard deviation of the values of the ocular wavefront error on all points of the pupil from a mathematical point of view. The PV (Peak-to-Valley) index is the difference between the two points of maximum and minimum height of the wavefront measured. Among the indices for the image plane, PSF indicates how the image of a luminous dot is modified on the retina when it crosses the optical media of the eye examined (Figure 2-8). It stands to reason that, on the basis of the type and quantity of the optical aberrations present in the eye examined, there may be an infinite number of PSFs present. The Strehl ratio is a measurement correlated to PSF. It expresses the relationship between the real luminous intensity of the object-image and the maximum intensity of the focal point limited by diffraction alone; a value between 0 and 1 is presumed.

OTF provides an expression of the quality of the retinal image on the basis of how vision of a grid is modified. The sinusoidal grid is an extremely useful tool in optics because it has the unique property of producing images with the same shape. In other words, a sinusoidal grid forms sinusoidal images of the same frequency (expressed in cycles/degrees) and with the same orientation. The grid, therefore, simplifies the specification of the effect of the optical system in just two parameters: spatial contrast and the spatial phase. OTF can be split into two further indices: modulation transfer function (MTF) and phase transfer function (PTF). MTF expresses the relationship between the contrast of the object grid image and the retinal grid image, while PTF is equivalent to the phase difference between the object image and the retinal image. These two components of OTF (MTF and PTF) depend on the pupil diameter. The improvement in the OTF, with the optical aberrations removed, increases the contrast and the spatial resolution of the retinal image. In a healthy visual system, this improvement in the quality of the retinal image is translated into greater contrast (with an increase in MTF) and sharper definition (with a reduction in PTF).

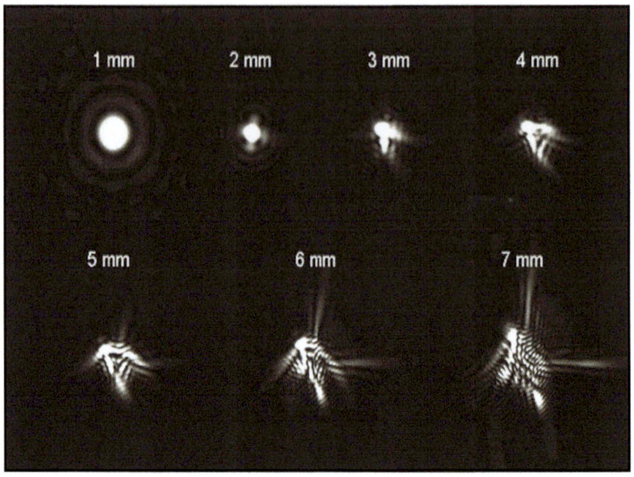

Figure 2-8. Point Spread Function (PSF) for pupils of various diameter. The optic aberrations are in direct proportion to the increase in the pupil diameter. For smaller pupils, diffraction represents the aberration that limits vision quality.

Biomechanics of the Cornea

The cornea has two main functions: it is necessary for the transmission of light, and it provides mechanical stability. Knowledge about these two issues is fundamental for refractive surgery. Manipulation of the cornea's structural integrity will result in a change in its shape, and this will influence the cornea's refractive properties. Quantification of the change in the corneal shape has been possible thanks to the development and use of a corneal topographer. The ultrastructure of the cornea has been accurately described in detail; however, the mechanical role of each part of the cornea has not been totally clarified.

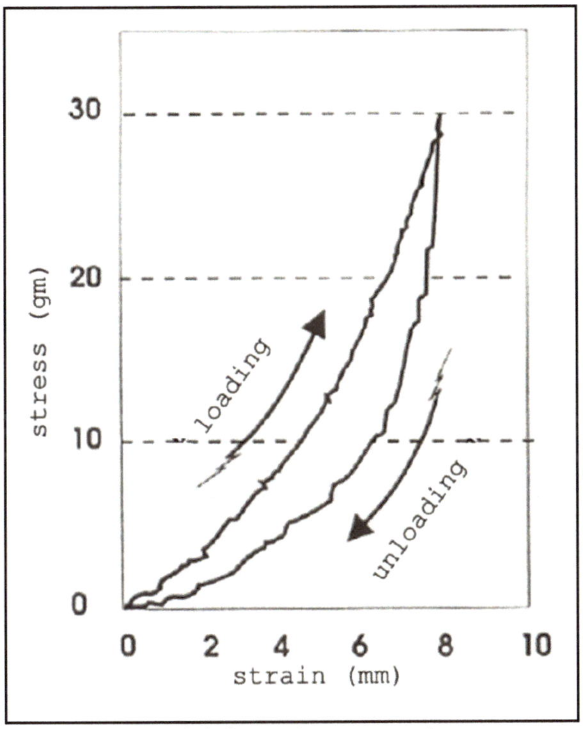

Figure 2-9. Load/deformation curve of an extraocular muscle. The area between the curves of extension and relaxation corresponds to hysteresis.

Biorheology of the Human Cornea

Rheology is a science that examines the force/deformation ratio in bodies, predicting how a material will behave under specific conditions. The soft biological tissues—cornea, sclera, and extraocular muscles—demonstrate a complex work/deformation relationship that is aptly illustrated in the load/deformation of an extraocular muscle (Figure 2-9). The soft biological tissues show a nonlinear work/deformation relationship and deformation curve of tissue subjected to pressure that is different from the relaxation curve when the pressure is released. This phenomenon is called *hysteresis.* Young's modulus is less successfully applied to biological tissues because the relationship between force and deformation is nonlinear. However, a series of approximate values of Young's modulus can be calculated at different levels of force (Figure 2-10). This linear approximation can be the instantaneous inclination (the tangential modulus) or a connection between two points on the curve (secant modulus). We see that the tangential modulus and the secant modulus are equivalent in the reduction of the approximate distance by observing Figure 2-10. The viscoelastic properties of a substance can be measured with the *creep test,* subjecting the tissue to constant pressure and measuring the extension over time (Figure 2-11).

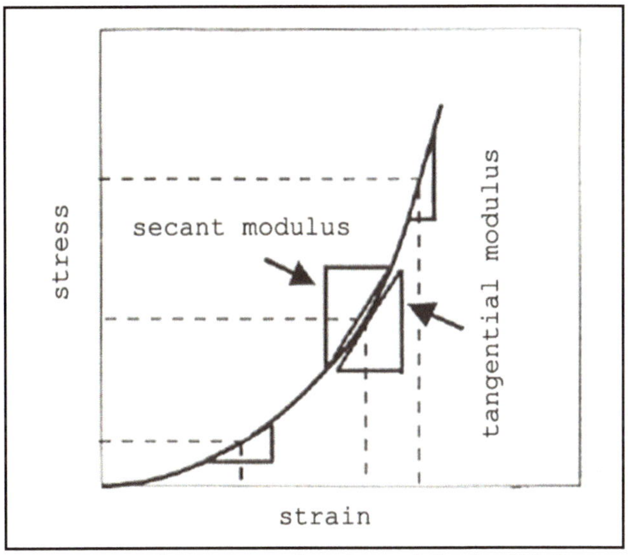

Figure 2-10. Linear approximations of the load/deformation curves for the nonlinear mechanical responses.

Mathematical Model for Corneal Behavior

During the development of the radial keratectomy technique, Fyodorov calculated a series of algorithms to predict the effect of this procedure and indirectly indicate how the cornea would behave. Despite the fact that numerous closed mathematical models have been proposed to predict the behavior of various procedures on the cornea, as we are referring to a complex system, it is not surprising that their reliability is limited by the complexity of the cornea itself. Iterative or open solutions, which can now be processed with the use of a computer, are much more useful in the prediction of real behavior, such as the mechanical engineering of complex structures. The stroma has the greatest influence on the cornea's mechanical response to pressure or stress. The weight of the stroma consists of 80% water, 15% collagen, and 5% other proteins, proteoglycans, and salts. The living human cornea is extremely porous, and it rapidly absorbs liquids. The microstructure of most of the stroma consists of 300 to 500 collagen lamellae embedded in a matrix of proteoglycans and water. Studies of the corneal microstructure have demonstrated its enormous heterogeneity. In the posterior two-thirds of the stroma, the lamellae are positioned parallel to the corneal surface, in such a way that every lamella forms an angle with the adjacent anterior and posterior lamellae. Anteriorly, the lamellae are oriented in a less orderly manner (and are often oblique with respect to the ocular surface) and are more branched and entangled with each other. This entanglement of the collagen fibers is more accentuated in the peripheral areas as opposed to the center.

It is important to investigate and analyze the nature of the inter-lamellar cohesive forces as the biomechanical model would suggest that the interlamellar connections determine a mechanical connection between the peripheral expansion and the central flattening that is observed following photoablation. Maurice and Monroe measured the force necessary to separate a sample of rabbit corneal stroma on a plane parallel to the anterior and posterior surfaces at a depth of 50%.[73] The force did not vary significantly in the various corneal regions. Smolek and McCarey performed similar experiments on the horizontal meridian of 16 human eye bank corneas and found lower rigidity in the central stroma with respect to the peripheral stroma.[74] These measurements are compatible with the histological observations reported above, which describe a more obvious entanglement of the fibrils in the peripheral corneal areas. Smolek, in further studies, revealed important anatomical-functional differences between the superior and inferior regions of the stroma.[75]

A distinction must be made between the cohesive forces and the resistance to sliding, as the two terms are often used incorrectly. The cohesive force is defined as the force necessary to separate a stromal sample along a cleavage plane parallel to the axis of the lamellae by exerting traction perpendicular to the cleavage plane itself. The cohesive force is therefore a measurement of the lamellar resistance to transversal separation. The resistance to sliding appears to oppose the sliding of a lamella over another one on a plane parallel to the lamellar axis (longitudinal direction). It is, therefore, an integrated function of the connective forces present across the entire lamellar interface and is presumably greater than the cohesive force (Figure 2-12). It is likely that both forces contribute to the displacement of the traction stress from the peripheral areas to the center of the cornea, as proposed by the biomechanical model of the corneal response to laser ablation (Figure 2-13).

The organization of the lamella in the stroma, and the capacity this collagen network has to support a specific load, is the logical starting point for biomechanical models of curvature variations. We often ignore the correlation between the interfibrillary constituents of the stroma and water, the largest component of the stroma. Collagen fibers are embedded in a matrix of glycosaminoglycans, such as keratin sulfate and chondroitin sulfate, with varying degrees of sulfation. Both of these substances, chondroitin

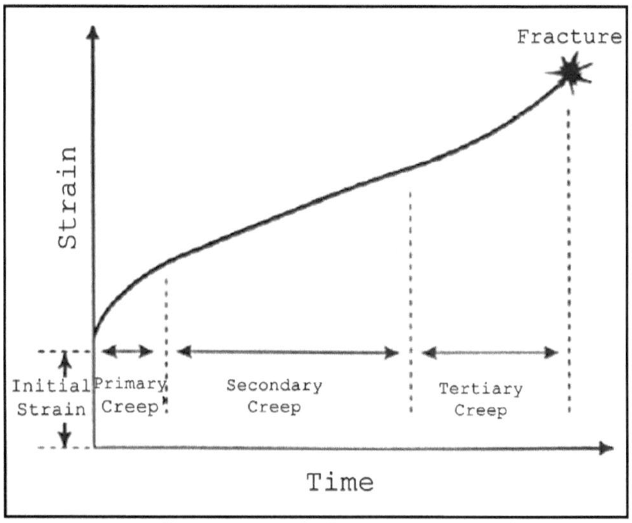

Figure 2-11. Illustration of three sections of a typical creep curve where the load is constant.

in particular, have strong hydrophilic properties and create negative intrastromal pressure that compresses the entire stroma quite considerably. The intraocular pressure further compresses the stroma through a direct effect on the posterior surface of the cornea and contributes therefore to the tension in the lamellae. The intrastromal pressure, frequently called "fluid absorption pressure" because of its tendency to draw water into the stromal matrix, can be measured by various *in vitro* and *in vivo* techniques. Its value lies at around -50 to -60 mm Hg.[76] Under physiological conditions, this tendency to hydration is controlled by many factors, such as lamellar tension, evaporation of the lacrimal film, the scarce permeability of the endothelial and epithelial layers to water, and the active transport of bicarbonates by the endothelium. All these factors contribute to maintaining the hydric homeostasis of the cornea.

The anterior stroma is less hydrated (3.04 g water/g of dehydrated cornea) with respect to the posterior stroma (3.85 g water/g of dehydrated cornea), and for this reason the hydration properties can differ throughout the corneal thickness. Katsube and colleagues[77,78] developed a corneal model and presented it as a series of thin layers that are consistent and permeable and interspaced with thick layers. They are soft and extremely porous (totally saturated with water). There is a negative pressure inside these layers. In the simulation of a corneal ablation, the first superficial layers are removed, and the negative pressure in the first porous layer is lost. This model justifies the increase in the peripheral thickness associated with corneal flattening.

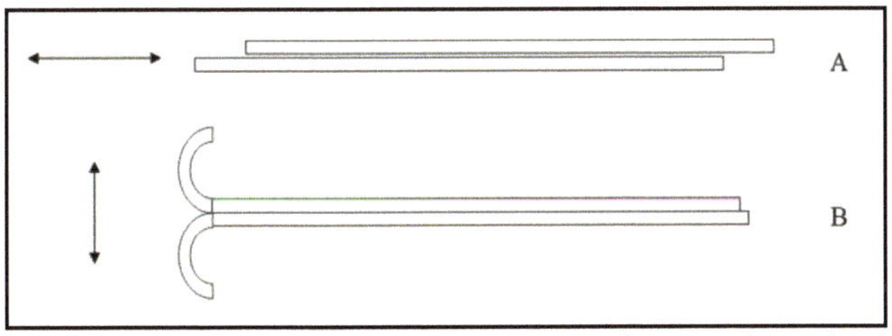

Figure 2-12. Diagram showing the forces described in the text. (A) Interlamellar resistance to sliding. (B) Interlamellar cohesion forces.

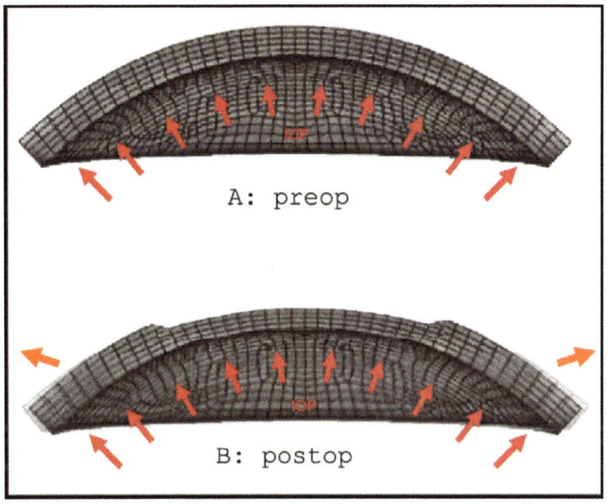

Figure 2-13. A biomechanical model of a cornea to predict the acute central flattening in the photoablation. In the preoperative period, the cornea is a stratified structure consisting of lamellas stretched from limbus to limbus with their curves maintained by the intraocular pressure. In the postoperative period, a certain quantity of lamellas are cut circumferentially. Central ablation reduces the tension in the residual peripheral segments of the lamella.

The Biomechanical Response of the Cornea to Photoablation

The cornea's acute biomechanical response is primarily linked to the stroma. The stromal layers develop tension that is limited by the traction of the extraocular muscles and the intraocular pressure because of their extension along the entire length of the cornea and their continuity with the corneal-stromal limbus. The hydration and swelling properties of the stroma are countered by the lamellar layers, the metabolic activity of the endothelium, and the compressive effect of the lamellar tension. The thickness of the stroma is associated with its ability to hydrate and is also an indication of its metabolic state. It has been suggested that when the tension in the lamellae is interrupted by a central ablation, the peripheral sections of the lamella relax and their resistance to swelling is reduced. The peripheral cornea then becomes swollen, and new traction forces exerted on the central cornea will cause it to flatten. As shown in Figure 2-14, the flattening of the central cornea is correlated with an increase in the peripheral thickness. The biomechanical model demonstrates how acute central flattening following ablation is accompanied by an increase in the peripheral thickness.

In the research for the ideal corneal ablation, one of the main problems is that the models used are inappropriate. These were developed initially to predict the corneal response to ablation.[79] In fact, the shape of the initial ablation profiles were based on a "closed box approach"; connecting the input variables (ablation algorithms) to the output variables (refractive defect, visual acuity, higher-order aberrations, patient satisfaction...) and did not consider the intrinsic biomechanical response of the cornea.

Initially, the ablation and the surgical results are correlated on two levels:

1. A cause-effect relationship dictated by the physical reality.
2. A statistical relationship defined by the retrospective analysis of the regression of the same variables in large-scale clinical studies.

Initial attempts with photorefractive keratectomy (PRK) exploited a simple ablation model developed by Munnerlyn and colleagues. These researchers presented an elegant analysis of how the shape of the cornea could be modified to correct both myopia and hyperopia. This geometric approach could be imagined as a *shape subtraction model,* where the tissue is removed with the laser to produce a surface of desired curvature. The cornea was considered a lens of inert material that could be modeled into an ideal functional shape. Munnerlyn's approach proved to be successful in the correction of spherical and cylindrical defects in the majority of patients. Nevertheless, this model of ablation induced a large number of higher-order optical aberrations and led to the demand for "aberration-free" profiles. In order to further improve the natural visual performance and reduce the induction of higher-order optical aberrations, the concept of refractive surgery must be examined in an objectively critical manner.

Corneal lamellae are permanently cut by the laser. This changes the central shape and will be added to the effect of the ablation profile. These shape changes occur with myopic and hyperopic profiles in both PRK and in the straightforward preparation of the flap prior to completing the laser in situ keratomileusis (LASIK) procedure. Central flattening describes the procedures for myopia and produces an action contrary to the hyperopic treatment. The induced flattening is proportional to the stromal depth reached. The creation of the flap modifies the corneal structure as described in the previous model. The basic difference is that the lamellae are cut and not ablated. The postoperative corneal shape and, consequently, the visual performance depends on at least three factors: the ablation profile, the healing response, and the biomechanical response to the changes introduced to the structure. Only full awareness of the interaction between these factors can improve the predictability of the results. This has key implications in the development of new ablation algorithms and procedures guided by wavefront measurements and topography.

Understanding the origins of variability of the results is essential to ensure the success of the ablation with minimal induction of optic aberrations. The shape subtraction model is based on three postulates, which were examined individually in studies by Roberts and colleagues and which have been shown to be invalid. These statements are as follows:

1. Only the cornea inside the ablation zone is modified by the surgery.
2. "What you cut is what you get."
3. Even when there are variations outside the ablation zone, these will not modify the shape of the central cornea and do not influence central vision.

The first postulate can be invalidated if we critically analyze the post-PRK or post-LASIK topography. Outside the ablation zone, the curvature increases significantly with respect to the preoperative condition with the appearance of the typical red ring (high values of curvature) that surrounds the flat central area following a myopic ablation. Moreover, the elevation and the pachymetric values are increased outside the ablation zone. These findings are contradictory and suggest that tissue has been added in the peripheral areas. Variations in curvature appear in areas distant from the ablation area. In the differential pachymetric maps, as expected, the thickness is reduced at the center and increased in the external areas. The second postulate was shown to be invalid when the predicted topographical result was compared to the real values. Two important findings emerge: first, an excessive flattening of the central area and, second, a red area beyond the ablated area that corresponds to an unexpected increase in the curvature that was not predicted by the Munnerlyn shape subtraction model. The tangential map of the errors indicates less change in curvature at the center and a greater change in the peripheral areas. The third postulate leads to a question: How is it possible to record the changes external to the ablation zone that also affect the central zone? Radial keratotomy (RK) has demonstrated that the cornea is a biomechanical organism that can change shape without removing any tissue. If the cornea was a homogeneous structure and was similar to a piece of plastic, RK would not be successful as no biomechanical response to the incisions would be observed. With the advent of the excimer laser, much of this was forgotten. PRK and LASIK induce considerable biomechanical changes to the corneal tissue though in a different manner to RK. These findings have driven other experimental and clinical studies that have demonstrated the biomechanical link between the central and peripheral cornea following ablation. The depth of the ablation is closely connected to the central flattening and to the thickening of the peripheral cornea.[80] These results initiated the development of the cornea's biomechanical response to the laser ablation, a response that invalidates the third postulate. Changes outside of the ablation zone cause changes inside the ablation zone, with an impact on the visual result. The *in vitro* and *in vivo* findings to date have shown that the cornea responds biomechanically to the structural modifications induced by excimer laser refractive surgery. This response is correlated with the ablation depth, in a nonlinear fashion that is a function of the number of lamellae cut. There is biomechanical flattening at depths that do not violate the limits of structural stability (ie, no deeper than 250 μm of residual stromal bed). To what degree the final shape of the cornea is dictated by the biomechanical response or by the ablation profile is still being investigated. Awareness of the existence of important influences that affect the corneal shape in addition to those created by the ablation profile is of fundamental importance for the development of customized procedures.

Thus, the final corneal shape is correlated to three factors: the ablation profile, corneal scarring, and the biomechanical response. The latter two should be understood and predicted to achieve a true personalization of the surgical and visual result. The "shape subtraction model" does not predict all of the changes that the refractive surgeon normally observes following treatment with the excimer laser; consequently, the aberrometric analysis alone cannot fully predict the visual result. So what is the solution for producing an ablation with minimal aberrations? The biomechanical responses must be characterized and developed in parallel with the wavefront analysis. Through knowledge of the ablation algorithms, the biomechanical response can be separated from the changes produced by the ablation. Finally, the topographical changes can be linked to the wavefront data to characterize the shape of the cornea and its functional response.

Optical Aberrations

The Zernike polynomials can be described as follows:

$$Z(\rho^n, m\theta) = Z_n^m$$

where ρ has a value between 0 and 1, θ between 0 and 2π; m is never greater than n; and m-n must be an integer. The properties of the Zernike polynomial include normality and orthogonality. The Zernike terms are defined within a unitary circle, and ρ and θ are orthogonal:

$$N_n^m = \sqrt{\frac{2(n+1)}{1+\delta_{m0}}}$$

with orthogonality, every Zernike function can be manipulated arithmetically and recombined separately. Alongside the component that depends on the radial order and the component that depends on the Azimuthal frequency, each Zernike polynomial is characterized by a normalization factor.

Normality means that a group of measurements of Zernike functions has been arranged to make an equal contribution to the RMS of the wavefront aberration.

Notions of Mechanics

Many ophthalmologists are not familiar with quantities such as deformation, force, and viscoelasticity, yet these entities provide a detailed description of the cornea's mechanical properties. Methods and techniques have been developed to provide precise measurements of the quantity of human corneal tissue and the various mathematical procedures necessary for the prediction of corneal tissue behavior as a response to a given laser ablation.

Deformation

Every body or, more precisely, every continuous isotropic system subjected to stimuli will be deformed in proportion to the intensity of the pressure applied. The nature of the material and the physical and chemical conditions of the environment also play important roles. Generally speaking, elastic deformation will disappear when the pressure is released; otherwise, the phenomenon would be plastic or permanent deformation. Some materials possess almost exclusively plastic deformation, while others are elastic up to a certain degree of pressure. This would be plastic deformation to the point of breakage. Elastic deformation can be explained by considering a metal cylinder of length l, diameter d, and the surface area of the base S. If we subject this body to two opposite traction forces F applied to the longitudinal axis, we see the following:

- Axial deformation, the deformation is relative to the length:

$$\epsilon_l = \frac{l' - l}{l} = \frac{\Delta l}{l}$$

- Lateral deformation, the deformation is relative to the length:

$$\epsilon_d = \frac{d' - d}{d} = \frac{\Delta d}{d}$$

Deformation is a non-dimensional measurement and is generally expressed as a percentage. Understanding the concept of unitary deformation ($\epsilon = \Delta l / l_0$) is essential, as summarized in Figure 2-14, where the same pressure (P) is applied to two cylindrical bodies in the same material of different original length: l_0 and $2l_0$. The absolute extension is greater in the larger sample piece; however, the relative extension (ϵ) is the same for both bodies, independent of the original length (l_0 or $l' = 2l_0$). The relative deformation (ϵ) is a function of force (σ = F/S), which expresses the force per unit surface area and not just force alone (F).

Another type of deformation is *torsion*, a phenomenon created by the application of two forces of momentum $\vec{M}$, producing rotation around the longitudinal axis of the test piece. This type of deformation does not change the dimensions of the test piece, just

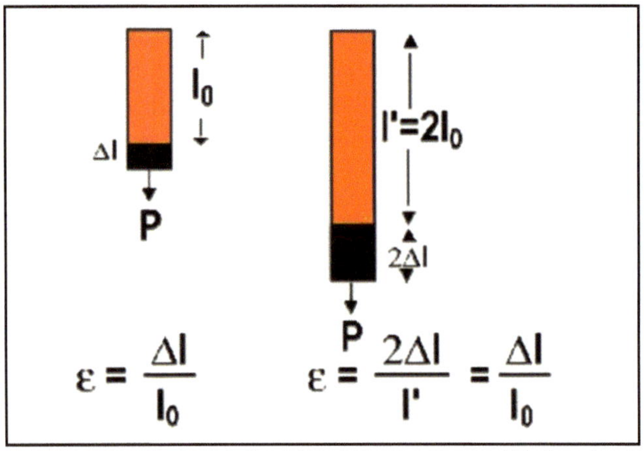

Figure 2-14. By applying the same pressure (P) the absolute axial deformation is greater in the longer specimen (l') however the relative axial deformation (ε) remains unchanged.

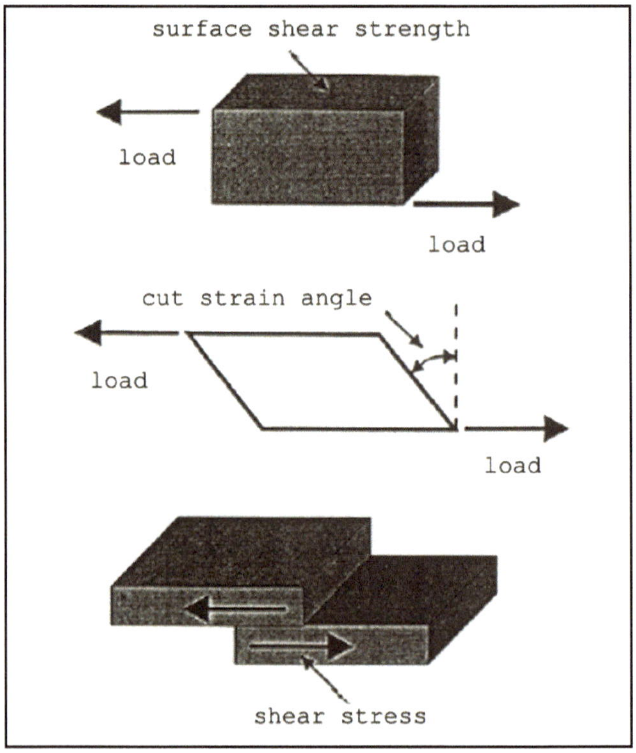

Figure 2-15. Force and deformation of the cut.

its shape and as such is called "the form deformation." A further form deformation is called cut or slide deformation and follows the application of two pressure forces (ie, force to two sides of the base of a cube). In this case, the form variation of the cube's volume creates an angle θ on the side faces of the cube, $\epsilon_t = tan\theta$, as shown in Figure 2-15.

Deformation can also be defined as *homogeneous*, where every volume element of the continuous system is deformed in exactly the same way independent of its position, and it can be defined as *nonhomogeneous* if the elements of equal volume deform in a different manner depending on their position. In terms of the elastic deformations, axial deformation (due to compression or traction forces) is expressed by:

$$\sigma = E \times \epsilon_l$$

where σ is the force, E is the modulus of elasticity or Young's modulus, and ϵ_l is the axial deformation. *Lateral deformation* is proportional to axial deformation, according to the equation:

$$\epsilon_d = -V \cdot \epsilon_l$$

where V is Poisson's equation, equal to 0.49 for human corneal tissue.

Slide or cut deformation, with the formation of an angle following the application of two forces on the test piece, is described as follows:

$$\sigma = E \cdot \epsilon_l$$

$$\epsilon_t = \frac{t}{G}$$

where G is the modulus of rigidity and εt is the cut deformation.

Nonhomogeneous elastic deformation, torsion, occurs following the application of momentum parallel to the axis of symmetry. It is described by:

$$M = C \cdot \theta$$

where C is the modulus of torsion and θ the angle of induced torsion.

If a rod of homogeneous material is subjected to traction and its length increases, its width will be reduced. If the dimensions of the rod remain within the final limits of the material, the ratio of pressure will be constant and expressed by the Poisson's value (υ), which is equal to

Poisson ratio = lateral pressure/longitudinal pressure

Mechanics: Force

In order to understand what happens inside a body subjected to pressure, the concept of *force* must be introduced. Force is defined as the energy transmitted per unit of surface *F/S* around a point, and it is created following the application of external pressure to a system. Force is expressed in "Pascal" units. In reference to mechanical resistance in terms of breakage of the materials subjected to the application of pressure, it has been observed that the greater the section of a given material (of given shape and

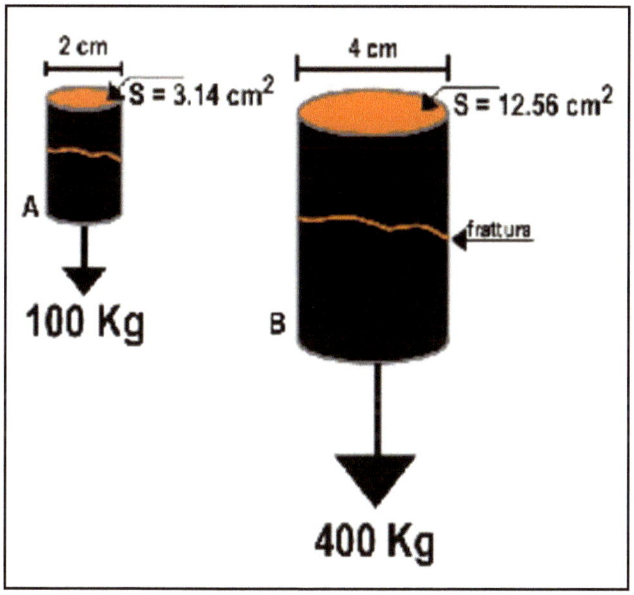

Figure 2-16. By doubling the diameter of the cylinder (from 2 to 4 cm) the weight to provoke the rupture will increase four-fold (from 100 to 400 kg).

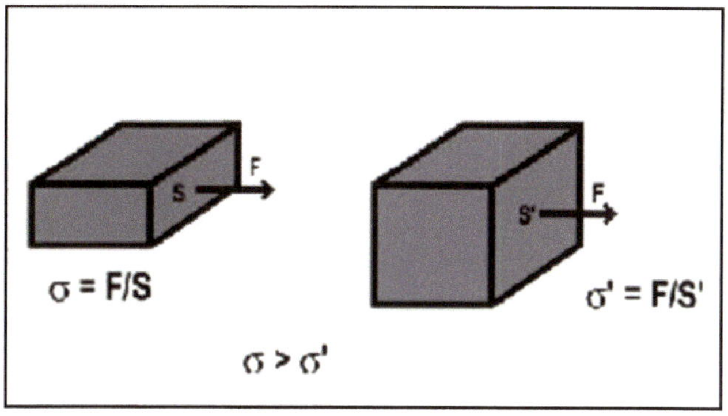

Figure 2-17. Solids with the application of the same force to different surfaces. For equal force, the pressure is greater on smaller surfaces.

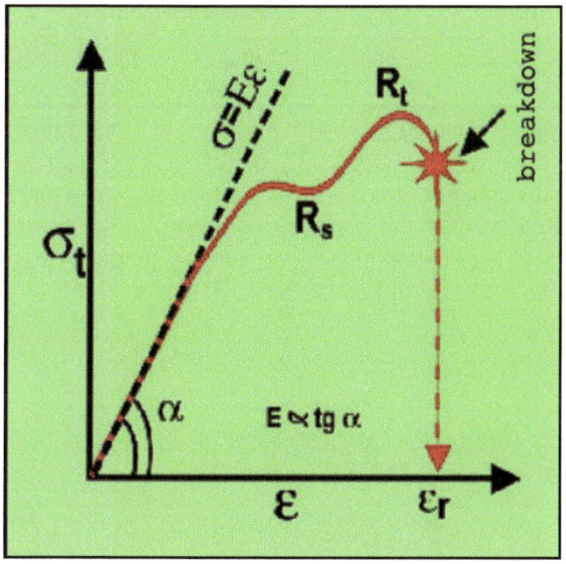

Figure 2-18. Pressure-deformation curve (σ - ε).

geometry, for example, cylindrical rods), the greater the force required to break the material (Figure 2-16). On the contrary, when the same force (F) is applied to two different surfaces (S<S'), the force necessary for breakage is greater ($\sigma > \sigma'$) where the surface is smaller (Figure 2-17). A "force-deformation" diagram defines the relationship between the applied pressure and the deformation of the material as shown in Figure 2-18. From the observation of a "force-deformation" diagram, it is possible to extract the constitutional laws of the material under examination. For example, in Figure 2-18, we can define the maximum force the material can withstand; in other words, the *mechanical resistance* (R_t), the *yield strength* (R_s), which indicates the force in the curve σ - ϵ that corresponds to a small "plane" of deformation, maximum elongation (ϵ_r) to which the material is subjected at the point of breakage *(fragile* or *ductile* materials are associated with small or large εr, respectively), the slope of the curve, particularly in the initial part where there is a directly proportional relationship between σ and ϵ, and the area beneath the curve σ - ϵ, which is proportional to the amount of work required to break the material *(tenacity).* In particular, the value of *E* (the slope of the curve on the linear tract) represents the specific rigidity of the material.

Mechanics: Viscoelasticity

Viscoelasticity is the term used to describe the properties of materials that show both elastic and viscous characteristics when they are deformed. Viscous materials deform in a linear dimension and demonstrate *shear flow;* elastic materials deform instantly when subjected to traction, and they return to their original shape as soon as the pressure is released. In elastic bodies, the force is directly proportional to the deformation of the material and is independent of the *speed of deformation.* The unit of elasticity defines the resistance of a solid material to deformation and is a property that depends on the material. In purely viscous materials, the force is proportional to the speed of deformation and is independent of the degree of deformation. Viscosity defines the resistance of a fluid to the irreversible variation in the position of the elements of the volume.

Properties that are typical of viscoelastic substances include *creep*, where the deformation of the body increases with time when the pressure is constant, and *relaxation*, where the force is reduced when the deformation of the body is constant. The rigidity of the material depends on the speed of application of the load. *Hysteresis* expresses how the force-deformation relationship of the material differs when the pressure is applied and when it is removed. There are a number of mathematical models that exemplify the viscoelastic response of a material. The classical models of viscoelasticity, such as Maxwell's, Kelvin-Voigt's, or the *Standard Linear Solid*, have been developed taking into consideration the elastic and viscous responses as two separate entities, represented by the spring and the damper (Figure 2-19).

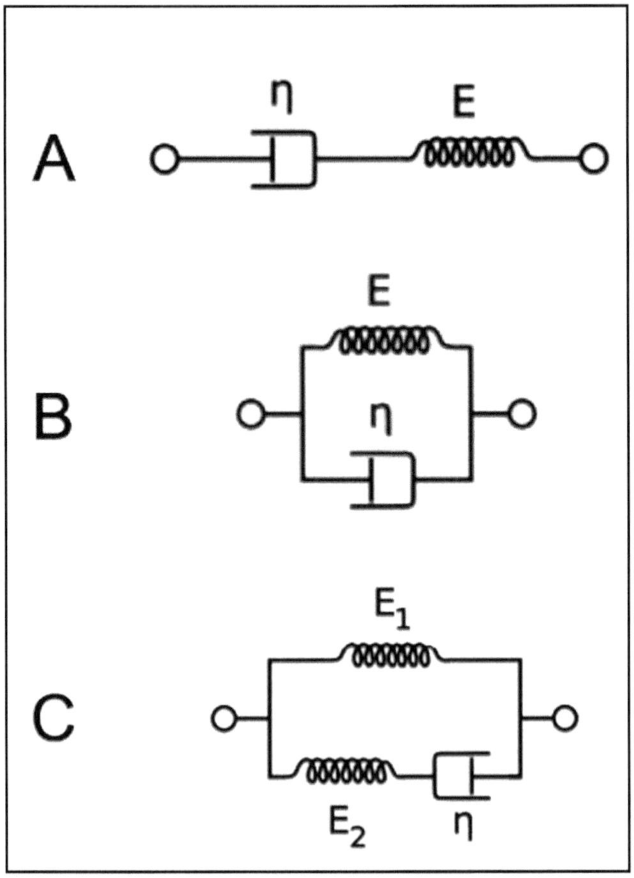

Figure 2-19. Classical models of viscoelasticity. (A) Maxwell's model, (B) Kelvin-Voigt's model; and (C) the standard linear model. Viscoelasticity is a mechanical property of the materials correlated to the speed and time of application of the load and it is modelized using a buffer and a spring as the basic elements.

Chapter 3

Photorefractive Keratectomy

Lucio Buratto, MD; Stephen G. Slade, MD, FACS; Sebastiano Serrao, MD, PhD; and Marco Lombardo, MD, PhD

Methods for Optical Correction

There is historical evidence showing that optical defects of the human eye were being corrected from 1200 AD onward. In the 13th century, spectacles were being used for the correction of spherical defects, and from the 19th century onward, they were used to correct astigmatism. Until the last decade of the 20th century, very little had been done to correct higher-order aberrations. Nevertheless, recent experimental studies performed using adaptive optical systems demonstrated a significant increase in the quality of vision following the correction of these aberrations. There are three main causes of blurred vision in the human eye: diffraction, aberration, and dispersion. The latter (dispersion) is considered to be a less important source of blurred vision in a young person's eye. Diffraction, created by the pupil diameter, is an important cause of blurring in miosis, reducing progressively with mydriasis, and is the only source of blurring that cannot be compensated. Aberrations are the main cause of blurred vision. Studies of the psychophysical aspects of vision have demonstrated that the maximum spatial frequency detectable by the retina of an eye free from aberrations is 78 cycles/degree (c/d). This would correspond to 20/10 vision on a Snellen table for visual acuity. The spatial frequency is lower for a pupil measuring 7 mm, lying at around 180 c/d. There is direct correlation between the quantity of optical aberrations and pupil diameter.

The spatial frequency that can be resolved following correction of the total optical aberrations of the eye is close to the limit imposed by the photoreceptor mosaic of the foveal area. It has been estimated that the distance between two foveal cones is an average of about 0.51 minutes of an arch or approximately 2 μm, which is the measurement of Nyquist's limit, approximately 59 c/d, or the maximum resolvable limit of the human eye imposed by the anatomical and physiological architecture. At frequencies above Nyquist's limit, the phenomenon of *aliasing* comes into play, a perceptive phenomenon responsible for the distortion of the images observed. In terms of optical quality, there are basically two criteria used to define the quantity of wavefront aberration present in an optical system limited by diffraction. Both are based on Strehl's limit ratio of 0.8. Marechal's criteria states that this condition may be achieved by an optical system when the RMS is not superior to $\lambda/14$. Rayleigh's criterion states that an optical system is limited by diffraction alone when the aberrations do not exceed $\lambda/4$. In order to achieve this optical quality in the human eye, it has been calculated that the aberrations must be corrected

Buratto L, Slade S, Serrao S, Lombardo M. ***PRK: The Past, Present, and Future of Surface Ablation.*** *(pp. 25-48).*

up to Zernike's fourth order for a pupil of 3.5 mm and to the eighth order for a pupil of 7.5 mm.

The maximum improvement in the quality of an ocular system may be to achieve the value of visual perception established by nature (20/10).

Nonsurgical Correction of Optical Aberrations: The Adaptative Optic

Originally, adaptative optic (AO) technology was invented to resolve the deterioration of images produced by telescopes and relayed to earth. The distortion was caused by the turbulence of the terrestrial atmosphere. The technological development was primarily driven by military investments, given the potential benefits of OA in making foreign satellites visible from land stations (and consequently open to attack). In 1992, most of the military information was declassified, which drove progress in every application, including astronomy and the science of vision. It was only in 1997 that the use of an ophthalmoscopic AO system demonstrated that this technique could correct high-order aberrations,[1] blurring, and astigmatism. The "Rochester Adaptive Optics Ophthalmoscope"[81] illustrated the potential of these systems by producing images of the ocular fundus of extremely high lateral resolution (approximately 2 μm). The foveal photoreceptor mosaic could be observed with clear imaging of the surfaces of the cones' external segments.

An AO ophthalmoscope consists of an element that measures the ocular wavefront, an aberrometer, and an element that corrects the optical aberrations measured, a deformable (or other) mirror with closed-loop system feedback. Figure 3-1 illustrates a descriptive diagram with the basic principles of the AO ophthalmoscope.[82] The ocular wavefront, originating from the retina of the eye under examination, will be affected by a delayed phase. The error of the wavefront is measured with a wavefront sensor. The appropriate phase corrections are applied through a correcting element of the wavefront once a computer processes the signal. The system works within a closed circuit loop. A number of wavefront sensors are available that detect the curvature, pyramidal components, etc. The corrective elements may be deformable mirrors, liquid crystal spatial light modulators (LC-SLMs), or deformable electromechanical micro-mirrors (MEMS).

The clinical use of adaptive optics may have considerable impact in numerous areas of ophthalmology

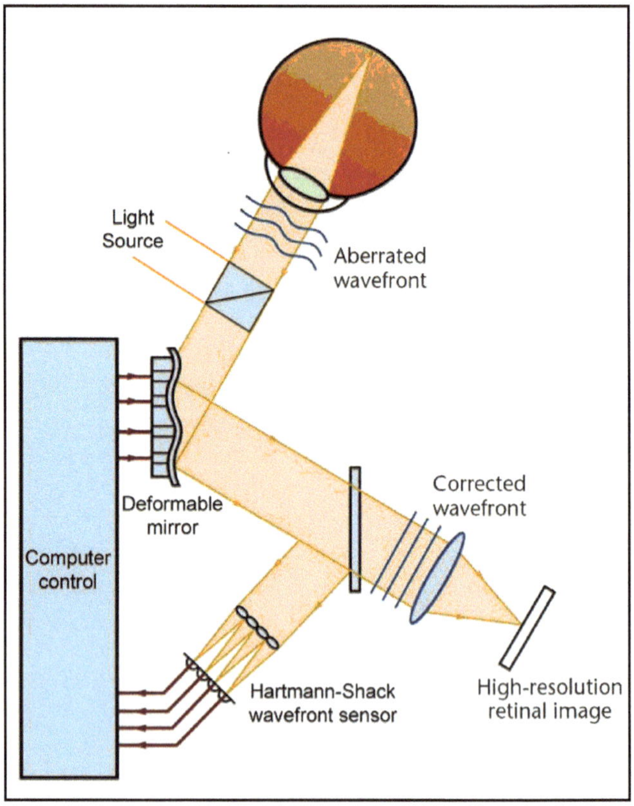

Figure 3-1. The operational mode of a system of adaptive optic ophthalmoscope. The system is complete with a feedback system: the computer processes the aberrometric map of the eye examined and transmits the compensation signal to the correcting element, a deformable mirror in this case, to the point of eliminating the eye wavefront error. Once the eye's optic aberrations have been corrected, the laser ophthalmoscope can achieve lateral resolution of aproximately 2 μm.

from corneal refractive surgery to the diagnosis and early treatment of macular pathologies of the retina. In actual fact, ocular optical aberrations limit retinal imaging.[83] The current systems for observation of the ocular fundus (ophthalmoscopes, angiographs, and optical coherence tomography [OCT]) exploit ocular optics as though they were objective lenses. This means that the image of the retina has limited resolution. The use of AO technology in the clinical situation can improve the resolution of the images of the ocular fundus. An AO ophthalmoscope can highlight early damage to the receptor cells of the retina (Figure 3-2).

Moreover, this type of technology can improve the imaging methods that are currently being used. OCT can resolve the images of the retinal layers to approximately 10 μm, so an AO system combined with the OCT can improve both the lateral and axial resolution (Figure 3-3).

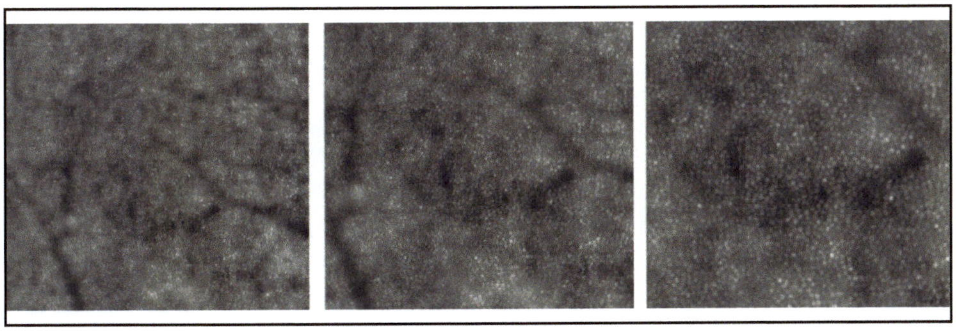

Figure 3-2. The adaptive optic ophthalmoscope permits the submicroscopic analysis of the retina. In the example, the photographs (at a range of magnifications relative to a patient with a healthy retina) show the photoreceptor mosaic of the perifoveolar zone.

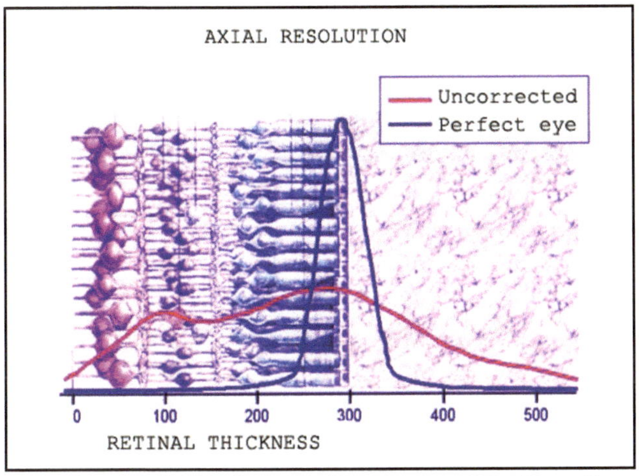

Figure 3-3. Elimination of the eye's optic aberrations may permit the visualization of the single retinal layers, without any overlap of the nearby layers, resulting in high-resolution images.

Another area of interest is correlated to the objective measurement of visual acuity. One particular system of AO can actually introduce any aberration to the vision of an eye, and this system is called "adaptive optics visual simulator."[84] By using this instrument, it is possible to test the impact of a specific aberration on vision. This may also have a direct influence in customized refractive surgery. This approach can also be used to scientifically study the impact of the different ablative patterns on spatial vision. Various studies have reported an increase in contrast sensitivity when higher-order aberrations are corrected with AO. These results would suggest that many people with normal vision would perceive an improvement in their visual performance if the defects are corrected in a customized manner, at least in a specific range of visual distances and particularly when the pupil is large. The correction of higher-order aberrations using AO systems has demonstrated a considerable improvement in individual visual performance.

Customized correction of the optic aberrations necessitates the exact determination of the ocular wavefront error and an accurate system of corneal ablation. The current excimer laser systems can remove submicrometric fractions of corneal tissue, approximately 0.25 µm with every pulse. This corresponds to a modification in the delay of the wavefront of 0.09 µm. If applied to the wavelength of visible light (550 nm for green light), in order to satisfy the Rayleigh criterion, the wavefront error must be less than 0.13 µm, and the excimer laser satisfies this criterion. Nevertheless, some inaccuracies, such as the profile or the ablation parameter and the biomechanical response of the cornea, can limit the potential visual benefit that can be achieved with laser reshaping of the cornea.

Excimer Laser Corneal Ablation

The word "excimer" is derived from the English words *excited dimer.* In chemical terms, an excited dimer is a diatomic molecule in an excited state. When it returns to its original state, it splits and releases the energy that was supplied to form the dimer itself. Depending on the diatomic mixture, different dimers are produced, and these produce different energy emissions, with different wavelengths. The mixture that is currently used by all commercially available laser systems to correct corneal refractive defects is argon fluoride (ArF) consisting of a halogen, fluorine, and an inert gas, argon. ArF emits radiation in the UV spectrum, with a peak at a wavelength of 193 nm, and the photon possesses energy of 6.42 eV. The energy of this radiation can break the carbon-to-carbon and carbon-to-nitrogen bonds (with an absorption peak at around 190 nm) on the corneal plane. This effect, where it is totally absorbed without transmission to the deep tissue layers, is called *photoablation.* The mechanism of photodecomposition has a reduced heat effect, and there is minimal coagulation of the surrounding tissues.

In structural terms, an excimer laser system (Figure 3-4) consists of a laser cavity, a gas tank containing the ArF mixture, a condenser for the emission of electrical discharge, an optic pathway for the transmission of the beam, and a computer that controls the correct function of the entire system and sets the treatment parameters. The laser typically interfaces with external devices to plan and guide the performance of the photoablation algorithm. The ceramic laser cavity contains the unit for the high voltage discharge (20,000 to 40,000 V) and is where the laser radiation is generated. A specific pressure of the gas mixture is maintained inside, and a ventilator fan circulates the gas to areas containing electrodes and ensures a constant gas exchange. The cavity and the condenser are the source of the laser beam. The maintenance of several atoms or molecules at a higher energy level with respect to the lower level, a state defined as "population inversion," makes stimulated emission more probable than energy absorption. The light therefore is amplified acquiring photons when it passes through a medium of gain. This phase is called LASE (light amplification by stimulated emission). The laser system is constructed as a system of oscillation, where the light bounces between two mirrors. The oscillation is maintained by the persistence of the excited "population inversion" state of the medium contained between the two mirrors. The laser radiation exits through a terminal mirror (this optic component of the system is subjected to greatest stress). The laser beam exiting is very uniform and is concentrated in extremely short pulses (between 9 and 23 nanoseconds). From the cavity to the corneal plane, the laser radiation is emitted along an optical pathway by a series of mirrors, lenses, and prisms and is subjected to changes in shape and uniformity.

The laser beam that reaches the corneal surface normally has greater density of energy at the center with respect to the peripheral areas. The *fluence,* which is the amount of energy flow per pulse and per unit of surface area of the ablated tissues, is optimal in a range between 160 and 250 mJ/cm^2. The ablation threshold lies at around 50 to 60 mJ/cm^2. Below these values, photoablation would be irregular and incomplete. The ablation is a complex and dynamic event, and the laser fluence drops with the depth in an exponential manner, as described by the *Lambert-Beer law:*

$$d = m \; x \; In \; (F/F_{th}) \; for \; F > F_{th} > 0$$

where d is the ablation depth by pulse, m is the efficiency of the ablation profile, F is the incident fluence of the laser pulse, and F_{th} is the threshold fluence for the ablation.

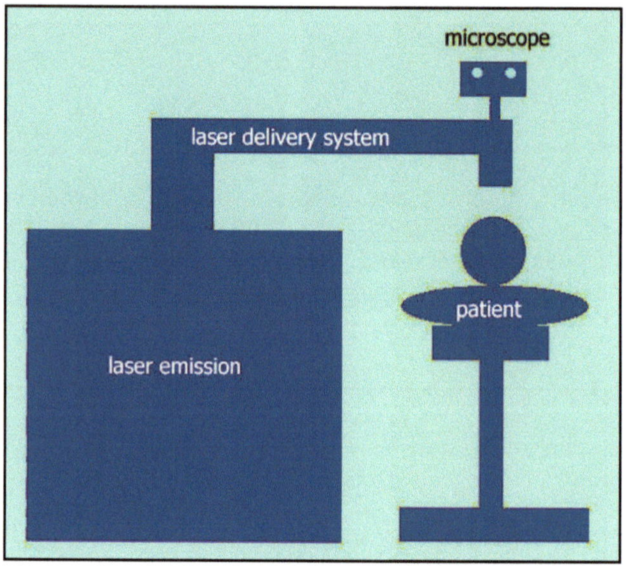

Figure 3-4. Basic components of the excimer laser system.

The *cut rate* is the quantity of tissue removed with every laser pulse. The current accepted value is 0.25 μm for almost every commercially available laser system. The *repetition rate* indicates the number of pulses emitted each second. It is expressed in Hertz and is an independent parameter with respect to the tissue. A higher repetition rate will produce a more rapid treatment but will heat the surrounding tissue to a greater degree (as the same area of tissue is revisited rapidly).

The laser systems exploit a variety of beams to model the corneal plane. The first available system was a *fixed broad beam,* with a diameter greater than 3 mm, and is now largely abandoned because of its limited flexibility, the irregularity of the ablated surfaces, and a marked inclination of the ablation edge. Using a spot of smaller diameter reduces the effects caused by the reduced uniformity of a broad-beam laser, probably because it prevents the barrier induced by the dust created during the previous pulses of the broad-beam on the corneal plane[85] and the overlapping of the impulses is more uniform. The scanning laser produces slit or spot beams. The *scanning-slit* laser has a rectangular-shaped beam that is distributed over the cornea with a linear or rotating system, allowing the construction of ablation profiles to correct every low-order aberration. The *scanning-spot* lasers can also be used to correct higher-order aberrations of the corneal surface. The small diameter of the scanning-spot systems provide a simple and flexible method for producing a complex ablation profile; the smaller the spot, the more likely it is to define a more accurate ablation model with fine variations in the ablation depth. Huang and Arif[45] simulated a series of ablation profiles with scanning spot beams of different diameter, demonstrating that pulses of diameter less than 1 mm and with a Gaussian profile can correct aberrations of up to the Zernike's sixth order in normal corneas, if supported by an efficient eye-tracking system.

Every commercially available laser device is fitted with an *eye-tracking* device of varying efficacy. These trackers reduce the irregularities of the ablated surface caused by movement to the head or the eye. The eye-tracking system is based on the recognition of the ocular movement and the spatial localization of the head and eyes with respect to an initial position. A tracker consists of the reception system and a system that repositions the laser beam within a specific tracking range (a radius of between 1.5 and 3 mm). A passive eye-tracking system determines an interruption in the emission of the pulses because of the movement of the eye that exceeds the tracking range and simply stops the laser, while an active eye-tracker system follows the ocular micromovements by centering the treatment on the exact position programmed at the start of surgery. All systems have elements of both passive and active trackers.

Surface Surgical Techniques—Historical Facts

The search for a surgical procedure that can correct refractive defects has driven the development of a number of laser ablation techniques. In theory, the ideal refractive procedure would be safe, efficacious, minimally invasive, adjustable, and reversible. Research has reduced the risks associated with this surgery, approaching it to the abovementioned objectives, without achieving them completely. In 1898, Lans described the concepts of keratectomy and thermal keratoplasty. However, a century passed before refractive surgery became reality. PRK was the first procedure of this new era. The first ablations were performed with broad-beam lasers and small optical zones. They were successful in many cases but tended to regress due to the irregularity of the surfaces and generate spherical aberrations caused by the steep transition of the edge of the treatment area with the untreated zone. These factors stimulated the need to develop LASIK. The ophthalmic industry thus channeled enormous resources and energy into the development of microkeratomes with high repeatability and minimal biomechanical implications.

Complications associated with the creation of the flap, and the risk of ectasia, drove surgeons to re-examine surface techniques and evolve them into advanced surface ablation (ASA) with the development of laser epithelial keratomileusis (LASEK), epi-LASIK, and smoothing and customized ablation. In recent years, the launch to the market of the femtosecond laser machines injected new energy into lamellar surgery, with the creation of thinner, customizable flaps (sub-Bowman's keratomileusis [SBK]) that are more repeatable in relation to the thicknesses. Refractive surgeons must consider all of these techniques as a complete and varied armamentarium to satisfy the surgical needs of all the diverse clinical cases. Evaluating the patients before surgery, on the basis of his or her physical and professional activities and the topographical, pachymetric, and aberrometric value measurements will orient the surgeon to one technique as opposed to another. Eyes with limited surgical exposure, corneas at risk of ectasia (low corneal, differential, and regional thicknesses), or patients involved in heavy contact sports may benefit from the surface techniques. Corneas with good thicknesses and patients in jobs that have little time to dedicate to convalescence may be oriented toward the lamellar techniques.

Dialogue With the Refractive Patient

An utmost important factor in refractive surgery is the relationship with the patient. The eye surgeon is faced with a unique situation in ophthalmic surgery: he or she is typically operating on a young patient in good health, who is actively employed and highly informed in the fields of information technology and computers, and who will research independently on how to improve his or her quality of life. For example, patients who are older than 40 years must be made fully aware of the concepts of presbyopia. A patient undergoing an operation to eliminate his dependency on spectacles will not be happy to unexpectedly have to wear spectacles for near vision postoperatively. The preoperative information must be complete and, as such, assumes depth of knowledge of the optical aberrations and corneal biomechanics. Being fully aware of the achievable objectives will reassure the patient. More specifically, the surface procedures will result in 3 days of discomfort (and sometimes pain) and 10 to 15 days of qualitatively imperfect vision; the surgeon must describe these possibilities to the patient and reassure him or her that this is normal and expected, avoiding any correlation of pain with a poor postoperative result or an operation that has not been performed correctly.

In the postsurgical period, the surgeon's knowledge of the normal topographical evolution and the analysis of the eye's optical aberrations will be the key in the relationship with the patient. A well-centered treatment, regularity of the ablated surface, which increases over time (Figure 3-5), and natural *visual acuity* superior to 8/10 will allow the surgeon to distinguish a good result. The objective data will allow the surgeon to give an opinion that is independent of the patient's subjective report, which can frequently be distorted.

Clinical History of the Refractive Patient

In some patients, certain general and ocular health conditions may be a contraindication to this type of surgery.

From a more general point of view, patients with metabolic diseases (diabetes for example) must be carefully examined, as these medical conditions can prolong the time necessary for the re-epithelialization of the cornea in the postoperative period. Uncontrolled diabetes with damage to the retina or other organs may be a contraindication to the operation. A patient with good metabolic compensation without damage to other organs can be considered for the operation following a full informed consent. The patient must be informed on the greater risk of complications in the postoperative period with respect to the rest of the population. Immune pathologies and abnormalities of the healing process, such as keloid formation and untidy collagen bundles, are generally contraindications to surface techniques and may orient the surgeon towards the LASIK procedure. Generalized infectious diseases, such as HIV, may be classified as contraindications to surgery.

In terms of ocular pathologies, the main focus should be on diseases of the cornea, followed by changes in ocular pressure, modifications of the crystalline lens, the adjoining ocular structures, the retina, and ocular motility. Generally speaking, corneal pathology is a possible contraindication to refractive surgery, and the same applies to glaucoma. In the event of opacification of the crystalline lens, the variation in refraction associated with this phenomenon

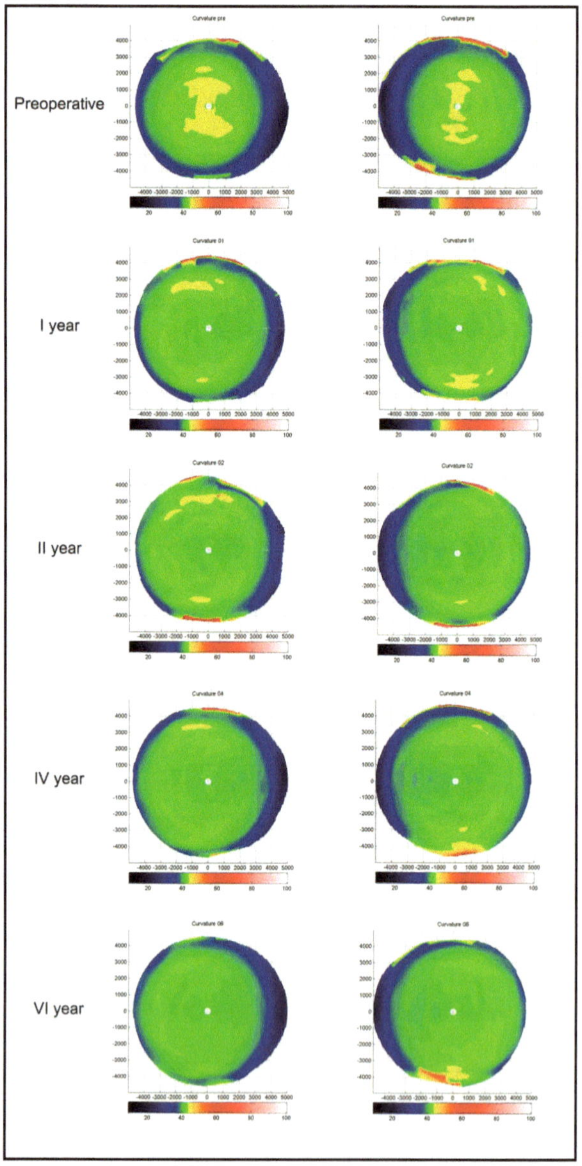

Figure 3-5. Topographical evolution over a 6-year period relative to a group of patients subjected to PRK plus smoothing procedure. The images show the mean topographical values of the population of eyes operated.

means that the refractive result may not be stable; consequently, surgery may need to be avoided. Peripheral retinal diseases deserve special attention, and in these cases, the refractive operation should be postponed, and the surgeon should orient his or her choices to a retinal laser procedure if necessary. In the case of myopic maculopathy or similar, the evolution should be monitored to avoid operating on eyes with serious reductions in visual acuity associated with foveal alterations. A consultation with a retinal surgeon is typically the right course. Significant esotropias and exotropias may need to be excluded from refractive surgery; however, later in the chapter, we will describe the contact lens test that may prove useful in cases of anisometropia.

Preoperative Examinations

The most important factor in planning the correct photoablative treatment is the accurate definition of the refractive defect. The surgeon must examine the patient and determine the manifest refraction and the cycloplegic refraction following the administration of phenylephrine and tropicamide. Testing necessary for the determination of operability includes topography, pupillometry, aberrometry, and pachymetry. Keratoconus or any other ectatic pathology should be determined and the patient properly counseled. Orbscan and the Scheimpflug camera can also aid with the definition of the thicknesses in the various corneal regions.

Ectasia is defined as the progressive curving and thinning of the cornea associated with the appearance of myopic astigmatism and a reduction in the uncorrected visual acuity (UCVA). Ectasia can occur as the result of the pre-existing corneal disease that manifests after LASIK or PRK or is hastened as a result of the surgery. In rare cases, the surgery on a healthy cornea can result in ectasia by cutting a flap too deeply or ablating too deeply. In any case, ectasia is a rare complication, and many surgeons believe that accurate preoperative screening can help largely avoid it. In 2005, a group of eminent ophthalmologists produced a document, the Ectasia Risk Score System (ERSS), which is based on the meta-analysis of retrospective studies to describe the most important and measurable risk factors for post-surgery ectasia. In 2009, Binder placed the ERSS findings into discussion by analyzing a group of 1705 eyes and re-opened the discussion on the essential points for the diagnosis of keratoconus or, rather, whether it is sufficient to consider age, topography, pachymetry, and the severity of the myopia as the only valid factors. The term *forme fruste keratoconus* is defined as a subclinical keratoconus, diagnosed only by topography that represents a patient at risk to develop keratoconus with or without refractive surgery. The findings supplied by Roberts in 2004 and Reinstein in 2009 defined evaluation criteria based on the differential regional corneal thicknesses and the curvature of the posterior corneal surface. These findings will transfer patients classed as normal by the ERSS into the high-risk group if analyzed by corneal tomography (Scheimpflug); moreover, greater knowledge of the biomechanical and physical properties of the cornea will improve the possibilities of determining the individual's predisposition to develop ectasia.

Contact Lens Test

At least three conditions can be helped with a contact lens (CL) test: severe anisometropia, irregular astigmatism, and monovision refractive treatments. Where anisometropia is concerned, normal binocular vision is often absent with consequent possible postoperative diplopia, and a simple test using a contact lens may exclude or confirm this hypothesis. Attention must be paid to amblyopic eyes, because with deep amblyopia the suppression scotoma is less valid. In the case of monocular correction, with undercorrection of the non-dominant myopic eye by 1.00/1.50 D, a CL test will be necessary to test whether the patient will actually be happy with this new binocular vision or not. A rigid contact lens can also be used to assess how much corneal irregularity contributes to decreased vision compared to scarring, haze, lens opacities, or retinal disease.

Evaluation of Myopic Treatment

Many patient selection criteria have already been considered. For example, a thicker cornea may permit treatment of more severe myopia and/or the use of wider optical zones. Treatment of myopia greater than 10 D is generally not advised, as a deep and prolonged ablation of the stroma can induce abnormal repair processes with lower predictability and stability of the refractive result. In cases of higher myopia, mitomycin C can be applied to retard the healing process as well.

Evaluation for the Treatment of Myopic, Hyperopic, or Mixed Astigmatism

In the preoperative evaluation of astigmatism, in addition to the exact determination of the degree and orientation of the refractive astigmatism, it is essential to determine whether the astigmatism can be completely based on the profile of the anterior cornea. The shape of the posterior cornea and, less frequently, the crystalline lens can also affect the amount and axis of astigmatism. In these cases, the patient must be informed that it may not be possible to correct the entire astigmatic defect with photoablation.

Another useful preoperative astigmatism evaluation is to define whether the topographical bow-tie shape is large or small, information that is considered in reference to the diameter of the optical zone for ablation. Finally, the procedure to treat the defect is chosen on the basis of the degree of astigmatism and the myopic or hyperopic spherical defect. In general, for astigmatism less than 1.75 D, the cylinder can be treated along with the spherical defect. It is essential to consider how the treatment of composite myopic astigmatism greatly increases the depth of the ablation at the apex of the optical zone, which might require a reduction in the diameter of the ablation itself. When the ablation is greater than 1.75 D, or in the case of mixed astigmatism, the technique of cross cylinder is recommended, which is described in detail in the section dedicated to the ablation techniques. When the astigmatism is asymmetrical, it may prove useful to perform the treatment under topographical guidance as described in the section dedicated to the customized ablation techniques.

Evaluation for Hyperopic Treatment

In the preoperative examination of the hyperopic eye, important factors are the amount of hyperopia to be corrected, the corneal diameter, the pupil diameter, and the mean curvature of the anterior cornea. These will determine the accuracy of the treatment. It is generally advisable not to treat hyperopia greater than 5 D, as the excessive ablation of the peripheral stroma can induce a biomechanical response, which can counterbalance the relative curving of the central region of the cornea and reduce the postoperative result. Modern excimer laser systems allow hyperopic treatments to be performed on optical zones of 7 mm or more and a transition zone of 10 mm or more. The treatment limit is therefore the maximum diameter of the cornea to be treated and the central curvature of the anterior cornea. The expected postoperative keratometry simulated should not exceed 49 D, in general.

Evaluation for the Treatment of Presbyopia

The correction of presbyopia plays a secondary role in surface photorefractive treatments. Nevertheless, some surgical strategies may benefit patients affected by presbyopia. Monovision, for example, is a surgical procedure in which the dominant eye is completely corrected for optimal distance vision and the non-dominant eye is under-corrected, by 1 to 1.5 D of residual myopia, to allow a return to natural close vision with less need for corrective lenses. More recently, ablation algorithms, used by some of the commercially available laser machines under topographical guidance, aim to increase the curvature in the central region of the cornea, increasing the spherical aberration of the treated eye and creating a multifocal cornea to allow the patient good distance and near uncorrected vision.

The preoperative evaluation of the patient must be completed, and the surgeon should discuss the risks and benefits of the operation in detail, customizing the treatment as much as possible to suit the individual patient's needs. For example, it is essential to give the patient a copy of the informed consent module based on the type and entity of defect to be treated, his or her age, and professional activity, etc, as well as the informative sheet describing the surgical operation scheduled. The informed consent form and information relative to the operation are updated versions of the forms distributed by SOI, the Italian Society of Ophthalmology, and can be found at the end of this chapter.

Surface Ablation Techniques

The preoperative phase is common to all of the ablation techniques. The patient is pre-medicated, and the skin of the eyelid and around the eyelid is cleaned carefully. If necessary, Valium or a similar sedative can be administered to the patient about 15 minutes prior to surgery. Once the patient has been identified and asked to lie on the operating bed, the staff checks that the patient is comfortable and that his or her position will not be changed during the operation (for example, arms and legs should not be crossed). Following accurate cleaning of the eyelid skin with Betadine, sterile adhesive strips are applied followed by the eyelid speculum to expose the cornea correctly. During the PRK technique, the epithelium can be removed using an Amolis brush or by instillation of an alcohol solution (25% ethanol for 20 seconds) and removed with a sponge tip. It is unadvisable to proceed with direct removal of the epithelium with a sharp instrument as it has been demonstrated how this action may produce irregularity of Bowman's membrane and may alter the refractive result. Prior to the ablation procedure, the treatment is centered on the patient's visual axis, and the eye-tracker is activated.

Following the ablation, a contact lens is placed over the cornea, as this will encourage re-epithelialization

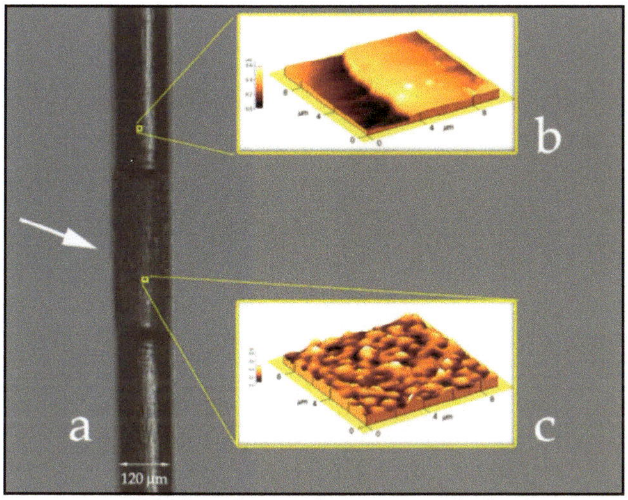

Figure 3-6. (A) The picture shows an optical microscope image of a human hair ablayed with a 2 mm spot. (B) The image was achieved with an atomic microscope in the non ablated region. (C) In the ablated region with micro-irregularities associated to thermal effects.

and will reduce ocular discomfort. The lens will be removed on the third or fourth postoperative day, or the time necessary for complete re-epithelialization.

In the days following the PRK procedure, the epithelium migrates from the peripheral areas toward the center of the cornea variably. The speed of migration is influenced by a number of factors such as inflammation, xerophthalmia, corneal denervation, the contact lens' permeability to oxygen, and the characteristics of the stromal bed. In order to define the speed of migration, some variables need to be taken into consideration:

- The density of the proliferative cells, situated in the basal layer.
- The density of the quiescent cells, situated in the more superficial layers.
- The concentration of all of the molecules that can interfere with cell proliferation and migration.
- Time from surgery.
- The geometric characteristics of the ablation.

In a normal cornea, the proliferative cells are equally distributed from the central region to the limbus. A large number of proliferative cells are found in the peripheral and limbal areas. The density of the quiescent cells is a function of the differentiated cells and the cell desquamation. Both growth factors and their receptors are involved in cell proliferation and migration. Standardized corneal photographs on PRK patients in the hours immediately after surgery have been done to determine the speed of epithelial migration and to investigate the relationship with the regularity of the stromal surface. The speed of re-epithelialization has been calculated as approximately 1 mm^2/h, and, as the area of de-epithelialization covers approximately 60 to 70 mm^2, re-epithelialization is usually completed by Day 3.

With the LASEK technique, the epithelium is freed from Bowman's membrane following the instillation of a solution of alcohol. The epithelial flap is delicately folded back at 12 o'clock, leaving a hinge attached to the peripheral epithelium, and following the ablation, the flap is repositioned on the stromal bed. Experimental studies have demonstrated that the epithelial layer is still viable following the alcohol solution application. The basal membrane adheres to the epithelium, showing that the separation occurs between Bowman's and the basal membrane. This shows the stability of the flap even following the manipulations necessary to expose the stroma. Preservation of the hemidesmosomes provides the presence of a structure that promotes the adhesion of the epithelium of the ablated stroma.

With the epi-LASIK technique, a special microkeratome creates a dissection between Bowman's membrane and the epithelium and results in an epithelial flap, which is treated like the LASIK flap and is repositioned at the end of the ablation.

From the evidence provided by research, it was shown that the rationale behind the success of the surface techniques is largely dependent on the regularity of the stroma at the end of the ablation. All the phases of the operation contribute to the regularity of the stroma, from the phase of the removal of the epithelium to the ablation procedure itself. Many factors influence the regularity of the cornea following the laser treatment: head and eye movements, the diameter of the laser beam, the uniformity of the laser beam, the debris produced by the ablation itself, which deposits on the stromal surface, and the heat produced by the ablation procedure (Figure 3-6). The irregularity of the ablated surface is the primary reason for a delay in the re-epithelialization and the remodeling of the stromal epithelium. Corneal irregularities following PRK give rise to three undesired phenomena: a reduction in the corneal transparency, a regression of the refractive result, and a reduction in contrast sensitivity and visual performance under conditions of poor illumination. All are caused by higher-order aberrations. Improved ablation profiles and the quality of the emerging laser beam have improved the quality of the ablated stroma.

The smoothing technique is used at the end of the refractive procedure to create a surface that is free

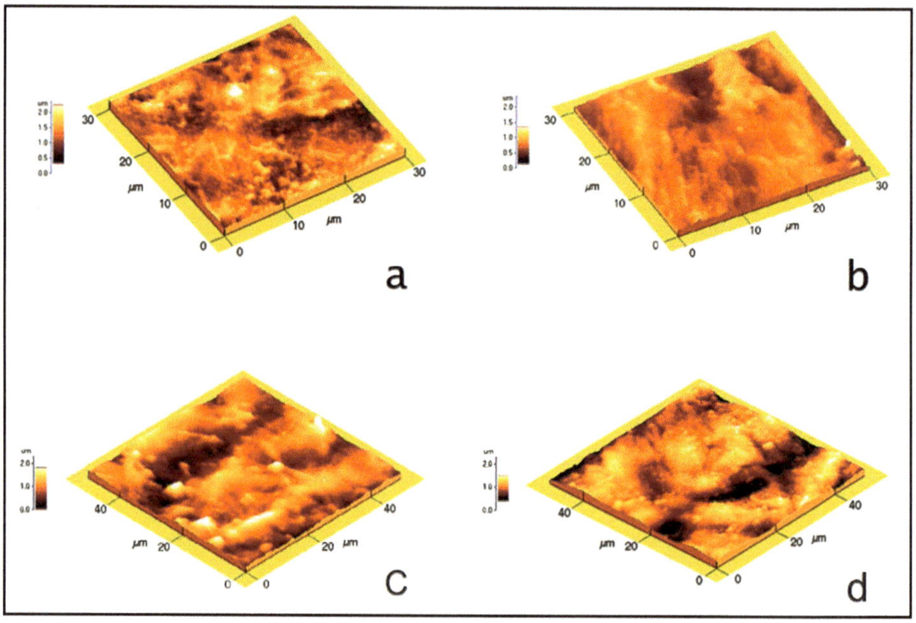

Figure 3-7. Images obtained with the AFM which show greater irregularity of the corneal tissue (pig) ablated with smoothing (A and C) with respect to simple ablations (B and D).

from irregularity (Figure 3-7). This technique is similar to phototherapeutic keratectomy (PTK), which has proved to be useful in the therapy of many pathological alterations of the epithelium and the anterior stroma such as Cogan's dystrophy, Reis-Bückler's dystrophy, and bandelletta keratopathy. The smoothing technique is performed at the end of PRK, using a viscoelastic substance (VES) that possesses suitable rheological characteristics.[87] The ideal VES must possess an ablation rate that is similar to that of the stroma (0.25 µm per pulse). The best agents have a viscosity that can form a stable, uniform layer over the stromal surface, coating the micro-grooves while exposing the protruding micro-irregularities to the treatment. A 0.25% solution of hyaluronic acid is the most suitable VES. The smoothing is performed with the laser set to the "PTK mode" for a depth of 10 or 20 µm depending on the algorithm generated specifically for the machine being used, with an ablation zone equivalent to the refractive treatment zone.[88] During smoothing, the 0.25% hyaluronic acid solution is distributed over the corneal surface with a blunt spatula. If the cornea is too dry, an additional drop of solution may be instilled and spread with the spatula from 12 to 6 o'clock and from 6 to 12 o'clock (with down-up movements), while movements from 12 to 6 o'clock (downward movements) are used to thin the layer of liquid: the objective is to keep the stroma covered by a thin layer of hyaluronic acid so that the PTK procedure is performed efficaciously on the irregularities that protrude from the surface. The laser system ablates the liquid mask and the unprotected stromal irregularities and will create a more uniform surface at the end of the procedure. A smoother anterior stromal surface ensures a more rapid epithelial adhesion and migration with earlier closure of the epithelium compared to an irregular stromal bed.[89] More rapid progression of the epithelium will lead to less activation of the keratocytes, less stromal remodeling, and less epithelial hyperplasia. The early and correct epithelial healing is the key factor for a better visual result, with less haze, less refractive regression, and less induction of higher-order aberrations. In experimental studies, *smoothing* has proved to be efficacious in achieving a more uniform ablated surface.[90] Ablations on pig corneas subjected to either PRK with smoothing or standard PRK have confirmed greater smoothness of the ablated surface when the liquid mask is used (PRK plus smoothing) compared to the standard PRK technique.[65,66] Experimental studies have also shown how the stromal surfaces subjected to smoothing have greater uniformity when compared to the surfaces subjected to the standard PRK technique. The improvement of the submicroscopic characteristics of the ablated stromal surface and the optimization of the laser-corneal tissue interaction are currently the two main themes of research in this sector in order to increasingly improve the optic quality of the ablated cornea.

Various clinical studies have demonstrated the optimal stability of the refractive and aberrometric results in myopic or astigmatic patients with PRK plus smoothing.[91-93]

Table 3-1. Complications of Surface Photoablative Refractive Surgery

Criteria of Severity		*Criteria of Time*	
Minor	***Major***	***Transitory***	***Permanent***
Hypocorrection	Severe infective keratitis (rare)	Pain	Hypocorrection
Hypercorrection		Fluctuating vision	Hypercorrection
Haloes		Haloes	Leukoma (rare)
Glare		Glare	Haloes (rare)
Haze			Glare (rare)
Mild infective keratitis			

Further findings from the research into re-epithelialization have shown how progression following PRK is asymmetric and the speed is greater in the temporal sector and lower in the superior sectors. These differences may be connected to the dynamics of the eyelid movements and with the different gradients of corneal eccentricity between the peripheral nasal and temporal zones. Another important finding is the greater speed of re-epithelialization following less profound ablations (up to -5 D) in relation to the less steep edges in the peripheral areas of the ablated zone and the more regular surface with respect to the elevated myopias. Clinical findings have shown better results in terms of visual acuity and refraction stability in eyes subjected to smoothing.

Medical Therapy

Medical therapy is largely topical with antibiotic eye drops administered until the epithelium closure has been completed and low penetration cortisone eye drops applied for 1 month. Artificial tears can be used after surgery, until the regeneration of the anterior stromal nerve complex has been completed. Oral nonsteroidal anti-inflammatory drugs (NSAIDs) can be taken for the first 2 to 3 days following surgery to attenuate any ocular pain that may be present.

Complications

The complications associated with a surface refractive surgery technique can be classified on the basis of severity (minor or major) or on the basis of time (transitory or permanent) as shown in Table 3-1.

Foreign-body sensation to perceived pain can appear 24 to 48 hours after surgery. The continual administration of artificial tears can relieve discomfort while oral NSAIDs may prove useful. A delay in re-epithelialization is considered to be a cause of all the minor or major complications of surface refractive surgery. The term "delay in re-epithelialization" is equivocal, as a minimum time for the closure of the surgical abrasion has not been defined. Kinetic studies on man have suggested that full re-epithelialization can be considered delayed at 84 hours. A delay in re-epithelialization activates a series of events at a molecular level responsible for the formation of haze and refractive regression, as described previously.

Under-correction is a complication that is observed in between 0% and 10% of the surface treatments, a completely different figure compared to the statistics of the 1990s, when approximately 40% of treated eyes required an enhancement treatment. The reason for the improved accuracy, predictability, and stability of the result is associated with the more uniform surface, which remains at the end of the photoablation treatment, performed with the most recent excimer laser systems, with or without the addition of postoperative smoothing. The simplest way of managing under-correction is the prescription of spectacles. Contact lenses can also be prescribed but they expose the patient to the risk of infections common to contact lens wearers. Residual myopia or residual hyperopia can also be corrected with further standard or customized surface photoablation procedures.

Over-correction can also be observed in the initial postoperative period. It is more frequently seen following hyperopic PRK than myopic PRK and will persist for 1 to 2 months after surgery. In mild cases, it does not require any therapeutic treatment; nevertheless, the patient must be fully informed of the reasons behind possible blurring of his or her close vision (over-correction in myopes) or his distance vision (over-correction in hyperopes), particularly in the initial postoperative period.

Haze is a form of opacity, of variable density, that affects the anterior stromal layers. It generally appears 1 month after surgery and reaches its maximum level at approximately the third month postoperatively, tending to disappear completely approximately 1 year after surgery. Haze following myopic PRK will appear in the central zone of the cornea, while following hyperopic PRK, it will be typically found toward the peripheral zones. Generally speaking, haze is not symptomatic, it does not cause a reduction in visual acuity, nor is it the cause of disturbances of the visual quality unless the haze is extremely dense. Thanks to the most recent ablation profiles and the smoothing technique, haze is now a fairly rare complication.

Glare and the formation of nocturnal halos are not frequent complications and are almost always transitory, limited to the first 3 months following surgery.

Infective keratitis can appear in the first days after surgery when the stroma is still exposed. It can be typically found in a peripheral position that does not interfere with sight. It can regress with no side effects or it can cause a corneal scar. It can appear as one or more infiltrates of the superficial stroma or as a stromal abscess. Therapy is based on topical antibiotics with the administration of a combination of broad-spectrum eye drops. If fungal or *Acanthamoeba* infections are suspected, the CL should be removed and stromal scrapings examined under the microscope. In the event of persistent symptomatic central leukoma, a PTK can be performed.

Some complications of PRK have more or less been eliminated with the new excimer laser systems, among them central islands and de-centering. Central islands largely disappeared with the use of small spot laser systems. Central islands are characterized by a small elevated area at the center of the ablated optic zone and can cause a reduction in visual acuity. PTK is the elective treatment for the removal of the central islands. De-centering is also a complication of the past thanks to the use of efficient eye-tracking systems installed on all modern laser platforms. It should be remembered that the best centering is positioned on the center of the pupil when the patient is asked to fix the luminous spot of the laser.

No clinical study has ever demonstrated the formation of corneal ectasia following PRK, except for form fruste keratoconic eye. Thus, it is important to screen out corneal disease before the procedure.

It should also be pointed out that the removal of the anterior stroma involves a modification of the biomechanical properties of the corneal tissue, which can reflect on a different reading of the ocular pressure following PRK with all the methods available today, both contact and no contact. Changes to the anterior profile of the cornea following PRK must be considered a phacoemulsification operation for the extraction of cataract, as the standard algorithms for the biometric calculation do not take the ablated corneal tissue into consideration. Nevertheless, there are numerous efficacious correction factors reported in the literature that minimize the error of the biometric calculation.

There have been no reports of significant differences in the incidence of complications between the various platforms of the latest generation of lasers, which have an ablation profile with an optical zone of treatment greater than 5.5 mm and a laser spot equal to or smaller than 2 mm diameter. Long-term results, with a postsurgery follow-up of at least 5 years, have demonstrated a significant reduction in the percentage of over- and under-correction, haze formation, and refractive regression with respect to the first and second generation of lasers used in the 1990s.[94] The frequency of enhancements has dropped from 20% to 50% to 0% to 20% following myopic PRK over the past 20 years, taking the various laser platforms into consideration, with the Technolas 217z and the Visx Star S4 giving a much lower enhancement percentage.

Enhancement Treatments

Enhancement treatments are geared to minimize the residual refractive error following photoablative surgery. The percentage of eyes retreated following PRK has been reduced considerably over the past 10 years, thanks to new characteristics and new ablation profiles. Enhancement treatments can be performed in eyes with under-correction or refractive regression. In the former case, the cause can be found in an incorrect preoperative evaluation of the eye's refractive state; in the second case, the cause can be found in an irregularly ablated stromal surface. The difference between the two sources of post-PRK residual refractive error is considerable. In under-correction, the surgeon can expect an excellent result following a standard surface enhancement; poor success might be expected in the case of refractive regression. The ablated stromal surface will not have the same ablation rate as the intact stroma;

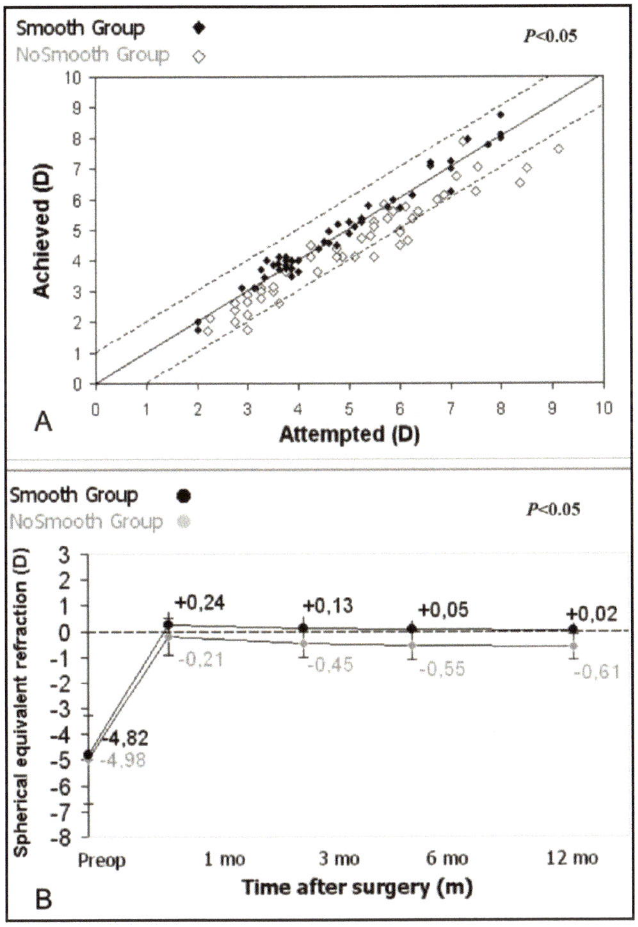

Figure 3-8. Scattergram and stability graph of two populations of eyes subjected respectively to PRK and PRK plus smoothing.

consequently, the ablation of the primary stromal layers was always lower than that calculated by the laser system. In the case of a uniform stromal surface, this phenomenon may indicate mild under-correction. If the stromal surface is irregular (as happens in the case of regression), the result is totally unpredictable and depends on the intrinsic characteristics of the ablated stroma. The patient must be informed that this enhancement is not a true form of refractive surgery but must be considered to be an operation that smoothes the surface of the corneal stroma that has already been subjected to an ablation procedure. Therefore, the enhancement must always be performed with phototherapeutic keratectomy with a liquid mask (0.25% hyaluronic acid)—a single procedure in the event of highly irregular corneas or as a second step following the correction of the refractive residual defect, in this case corresponding to postoperative smoothing.

Clinical Results

In 2000, Dr. George Waring, who was editor of the *Journal of Refractive Surgery* at the time, published an article called "Standard Graphs for Reporting Refractive Surgery" in which he described a series of graphs to represent the results of laser surgery in a standardized manner. Any refractive surgeon who wishes to give a detailed description of his results and compare the findings from his own laser center with those of other surgeons can express them using these standards. The graphs listed by Waring include the "scattergram" and the "stability graph." In the scattergram, the x-axis indicates the starting refraction of the individual eye (expressed in spherical equivalent refraction), and the y-axis indicates the correction achieved after surgery. The immediate vision results will indicate whether the surgery has produced under-correction, over-correction, or whether the results are ±1.00 D spherical equivalent refraction. In the second stability graph, the x-axis indicates the time (expressed in months or years) from surgery, and the y-axis indicates the mean spherical equivalent of all the operated eyes. The results will tell us whether our surgery has been stable over time or not. Typical findings relative to two groups of 50 patients operated by standard PRK or PRK plus smoothing, at 1 year from surgery, are expressed in the graphs in Figure 3-8. The scattergram of the expected refraction vs the real refraction achieved illustrates that 92% of patients have a spherical equivalent ±0.50 D with 100% of the patients between ±1.00 D from emmetropia. The stability over the first year shows us that, following a mild hyperopic shift in the immediate postoperative period, the result will likely be stable over time.

In order to describe the impact and the correction of astigmatism, which is not expressed with the scattergram or the stability graph, another graph called "defocus equivalent" must be used. This considers astigmatism independently of the spherical error and is significant when associated with the previous graphs. The most important and indispensable measurement is the loss of lines of best-corrected visual acuity (BCVA) and can be expressed using the *safety index*. This graph represents the relationship between the preoperative and postoperative BCVA. The efficacy of the surgical procedures can be described using the *efficacy index*,[95] which expresses the relationship between the postoperative UCVA and the preoperative BCVA.

The regularity of the corneal surface is expressed by two indices: Best Fit Topographic Irregularity (BFTI)

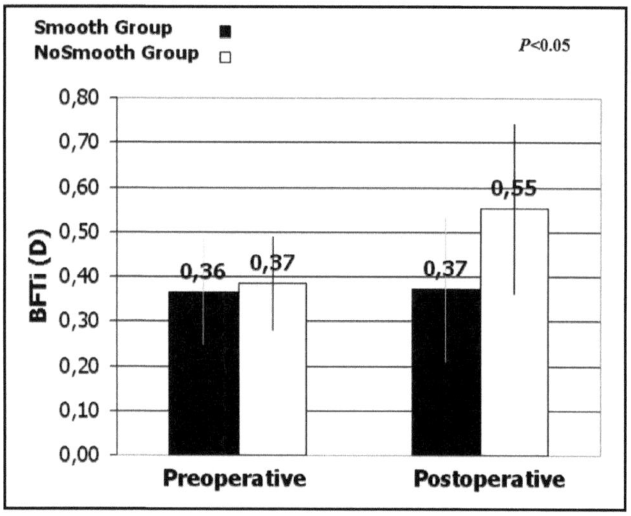

Figure 3-9. Indices of topographical irregularity in eyes subjected to PRK and PRK plus smoothing, before and after surgery.

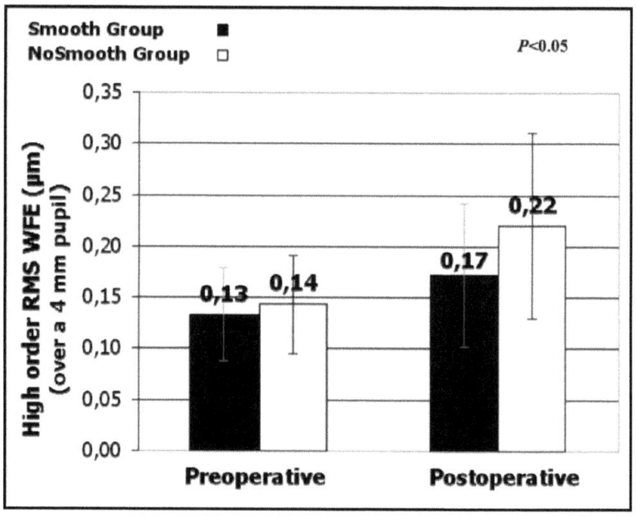

Figure 3-10. RMS of the high-order aberrations compared to eyes subjected to PRK and PRK plus smoothing, before and after surgery.

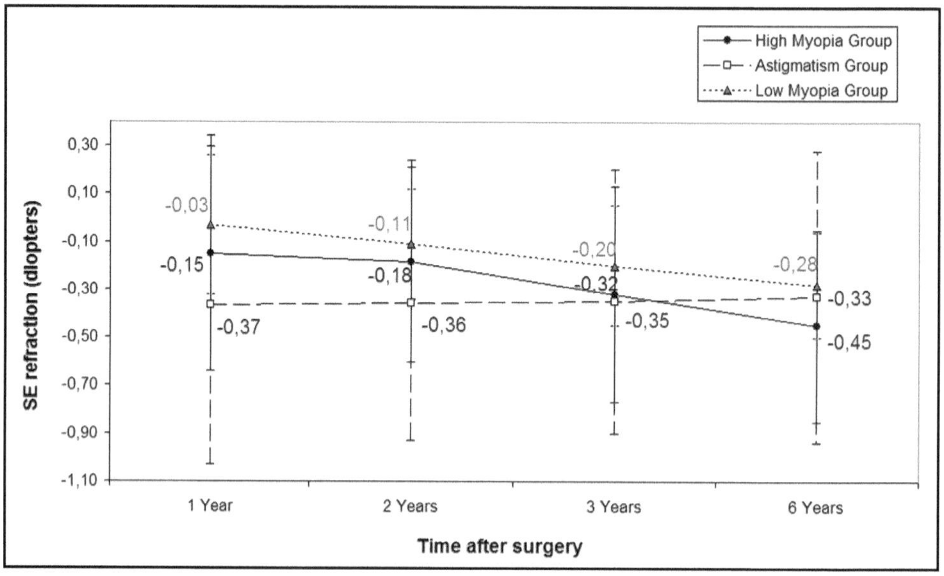

Figure 3-11. Follow-up of the spherical equivalent over a 6-year period for three groups of patients operated to correct mild, moderate, and severe myopia.

or Maloney's Index[96] and the total higher-order root mean square (RMS). BFTI is measured in diopters and expresses a mean value of the variation of curvature in the central 4 mm of topography, corresponding approximately to the mesopic pupil. RMS is the sum of the differences between the measured cornea and the value of spherical cylinder that best represent that specific cornea. The total higher-order RMS is expressed in microns and indicates the entity of higher-order aberrations of the anterior cornea. Figures 3-9 and 3-10 illustrate the values of pre- and postoperative BFTI and RMS, 1 year from surgery, measured in two groups of eyes subjected to standard PRK and PRK plus smoothing, respectively. The postoperative values are greater than the preoperative ones showing that the ablation increases the irregularity of the surface. In 18% of cases, there was a reduction in the total higher-order RMS that indicates an improvement in the optic properties of the corneal surface. With longer follow-up, a statistically significant regression of 0.25 to 0.50 D was observed over a 6-year period (Figure 3-11). There is no significant difference in the vision quality in daylight. After treatment, there may be an improvement of up to 5 myopic diopters. At night, patients operated for severe myopia may complain of halos around light sources; this problem is not serious and is less debilitating than the phenomena created some years ago when smaller optic zones were used.

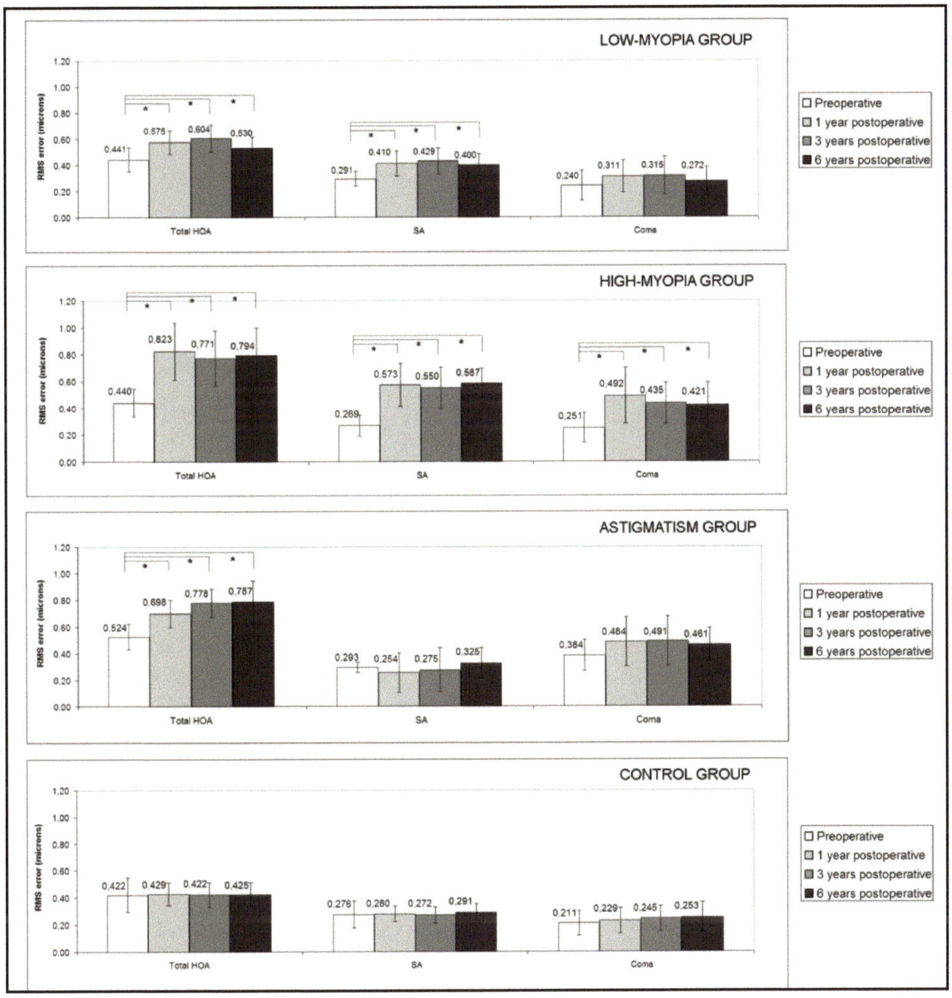

Figure 3-12. Six-year follow-up of the high-order aberrations, total HOA RMS, coma, and spherical aberration above a pupil diameter of 3.5 mm, in three groups of patients operated for low, moderate, and severe myopia. Bottom graph: The evolution of the high-order aberrations in a group of same-age patients not subjected to surgery.

The reference pupil dimension should be specified in the analysis of the results, as the severity of the optical aberrations is a function of the pupil diameter. The mean measurement of the mesopic and scotopic pupil in young adults is approximately 3.50 and 6.00 mm, respectively. For this reason, the description of the optic quality with daylight and at night must be referred to the relative wavefront measured at 3.50 mm and at 6.00 mm. For a pupil of 3.5 mm, the total higher-order RMS and coma will normally increase following myopic treatments in excess of 5 D. The degree of spherical aberration (Sa) increases in both the mild and severe myopias 1 year from surgery, to stabilize over successive years (Figure 3-12). For a scotopic pupil of diameter 6.00 mm, the total higher-order RMS and the Sa normally increase with respect to the preoperative values for both low and high myopias and will be stable over the years. An increase in total higher-order RMS is usually detected following an astigmatic ablation. Figure 3-13 illustrates the characteristic higher-order RMS over a 6-year follow-up period for a pupil of 6.00 mm. The significant increase in the higher-order optical aberrations has been measured with all of the commercially available excimer lasers. There are no significant differences between the various platforms of the latest generation in the increase of Sa[97] when the treatment has been performed on optic zones of diameter 6 mm or more. High-quality PSFs result from the measurements on pupils of diameter 3.50 mm in the ablations of both low and high myopias, and there are only slight differences observed between the preoperative and postoperative states. For pupils of diameter 6.00 mm, there is a clear increase in the effects of the spherical aberration on the quality of PSF, particularly where deep ablations are concerned (Figure 3-14).

Ablation Profiles

Munnerlyn and colleagues[98] were the first to describe the equation used as the starting point for the development of the current ablation algorithms. These

Figure 3-13. Six-year follow-up of the evolution of the high-order aberrations, total HOA RMS, coma, and spherical aberration above a pupil diameter of 6.0 mm, in three groups of patients operated for low, moderate, and severe myopia. Bottom graph: The evolution of high-order aberrations in a group of same-age myopic patients not subjected to surgery.

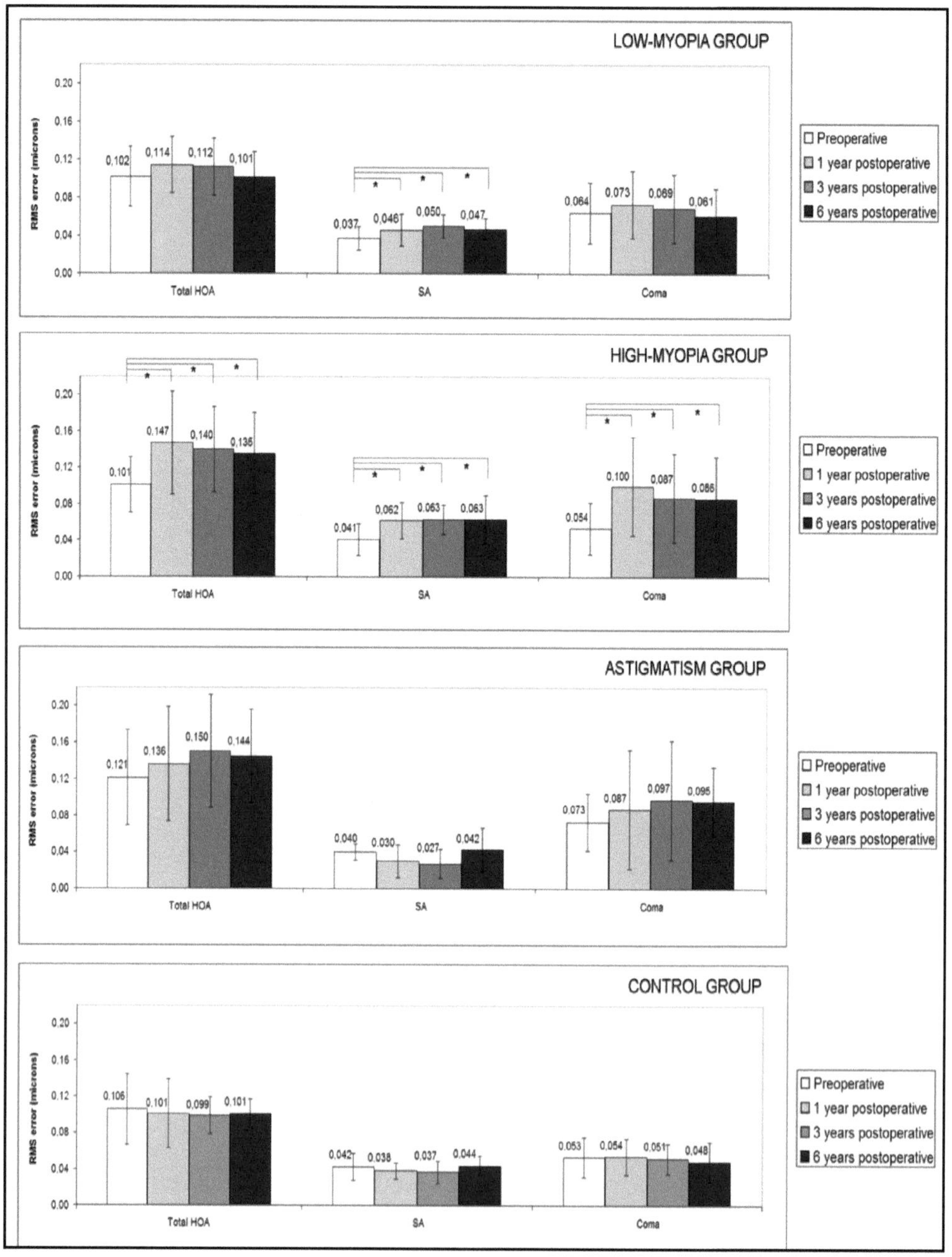

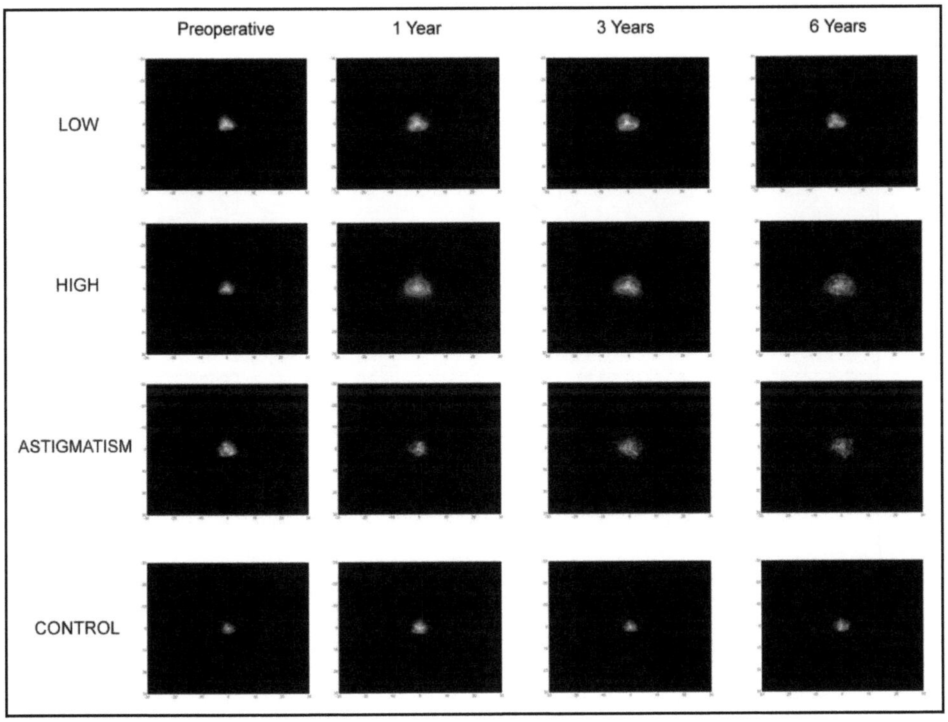

Figure 3-14. Mean point spread functions (PSFs) calculated for a pupil diameter of 6 mm in the same population of patients shown in Figure 3-13, operated for mild, moderate, and severe myopia. Note how the PSF is more defocalized following the treatment of severe myopia.

produced the profile of the ablated corneal depth for the models of myopic and hyperopic ablation:

$$Ablation\ depth\ Z_0 = \frac{diameter\ ZO^2\ x\ n°\ diopters}{3}$$

where Z_0 is the ablation depth at the center of the cornea and ZO is the diameter of the ablation zone. This derivation is based on the theory of thin lenses and para-axial optics considering the tissue for removal as a contact lens of diameter (D). In Munnerlyn's model, the pre- and postoperative corneas are considered as spherical lenses. The removal of tissue is therefore equivalent to the addition of a thin negative (or positive) lens of power Φ given by:

$$\Phi = (n-1)\ \frac{1}{R_{post}} - \frac{1}{R_{pre}}$$

where R_{pre} is the radius of preoperative corneal curvature and R_{post} is the radius of desired postoperative curvature and n has a value of 1.3771, the refractive index of the cornea. The thickness of this contact lens Z_0 is approximately

$$Z_0 = \frac{-D^2\ x\ n°}{8(n-1)}$$

Munnerlyn's model is called the shape subtraction model and considers the cornea as a homogeneous structure, like a piece of plastic. The shape subtraction model is based on three factors that have been widely described in the chapter on corneal biomechanics and that can explain the variability of the result and the aberrations produced by the excimer laser refractive procedures. Munnerlyn's model has been designed to eliminate the spherical-cylindrical refractive defects. The drawback with this equation is that it actually aims to correct the spherical error alone, ignoring the other aberrations of the corneal surface. In actual fact, it is efficacious in the regions where the cornea is clearly spherical in shape, but this will limit the efficacy of Munnerlyn's formula to a small area around the visual axis. Moreover, Munnerlyn's model modifies the degree of spherical aberration in an uncontrolled manner and induces significant visual effects, such as glare and halos around light sources.

Despite having natural visual acuity that is satisfactory for all of their daily activities, many patients who have been treated with profiles based on Munnerlyn's algorithm complain of a sight quality that is less than optimal under conditions of reduced environmental lighting, due to an excessive increase in the spherical aberration (Figure 3-15).

Various studies have demonstrated the presence of a large number of higher-order aberrations in eyes subjected to excimer laser corneal refractive surgery, with a reduction in the visual performance particularly under conditions of scotopic light, with the pupil diameter over 5.00 mm. In particular, from the analysis of the wavefront of the primary corneal surfaces subjected to PRK, there are two Zernike terms that involve the corneal aberrometric structure more than

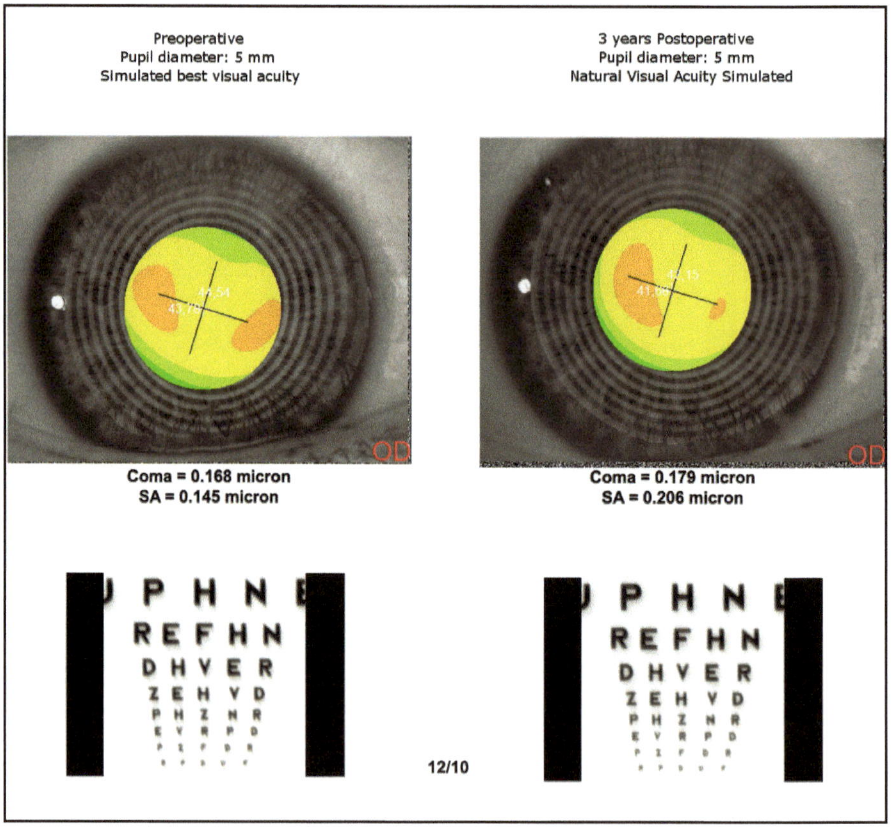

Figure 3-15. Simulated visual acuity of an eye before (left) and after (right) the operation of surface refractive surgery in the treatment of mild myopia. Three years from surgery, the patient's visual acuity is quantitatively and qualitatively satisfactory, there is a very limited increase in the high-order aberrations induced by surgery.

others, coma and spherical aberration.[99,100] It is also a well-known fact that the greater the correction, the greater the entity of higher-order aberrations induced by surgery. Analysis of the postoperative corneal aberrometric maps of patients subjected to excimer laser refractive surgery demonstrates a modification of the structure of the optic aberrations of the corneal surface (Figure 3-16). If we consider the aberrations for a 7-mm diameter pupil, there is a constant increase in the negative sphericity that can be attributed to the ablation of the central portion of the corneal tissue and a variable increase of the other Zernike terms in relation to the transparency of the corneal tissue and the uniformity of the ablated surface. In order to check the spherical aberration induced by the refractive surgery, it is essential to evaluate the aspherical component in the postoperative cornea. The first attempts of evolution of the ablations with a single optic zone occurred with transition and multiple zones (shape-splitting). Two types of transition can be identified; the first are simply added to the optic zone and are small or predetermined, unchangeable, and do not allow a real improvement of the profile in relation to the correction. The most efficacious transition zone results from an ablation algorithm that has been studied dynamically on the basis of the preoperative mean radius of curvature and the desired optic zone.

Through the multizone (shape-splitting) ablations, surgeons have attempted to distribute the treatment into increasing diameters with a fairly constant thickness. This will create a compromise between the ablation depth and the width of the optic zone while creating an initial transition zone. The splitting technique was developed to avoid the creation of an abrupt transition, shown by a topographical "red ring" in the middle peripheral area. The technique leads to the formation of optic zones that are larger than those programmed. The disadvantages of this technique were the difficulty associated with centering the zones on each other, resulting in de-centrations and irregular astigmatism, marked regression, and severe haze due to the inaccuracy of the transition zone. This was particularly evident when the transition between the various zones was not created and was subjected to a final smoothing procedure. In actual fact, multizones required the removal of the same amount of tissue from each zone with a different dioptric correction, thus creating an inconstant corneal dioptric gradient that was not gradual.

The correction of astigmatism according to Munnerlyn's algorithm has been frequently affected by regression, haze, and visual disturbances. There is general agreement that these complications are due to the transition between the nonablated peripheral portion and ablated corneal surface. The algorithm involves

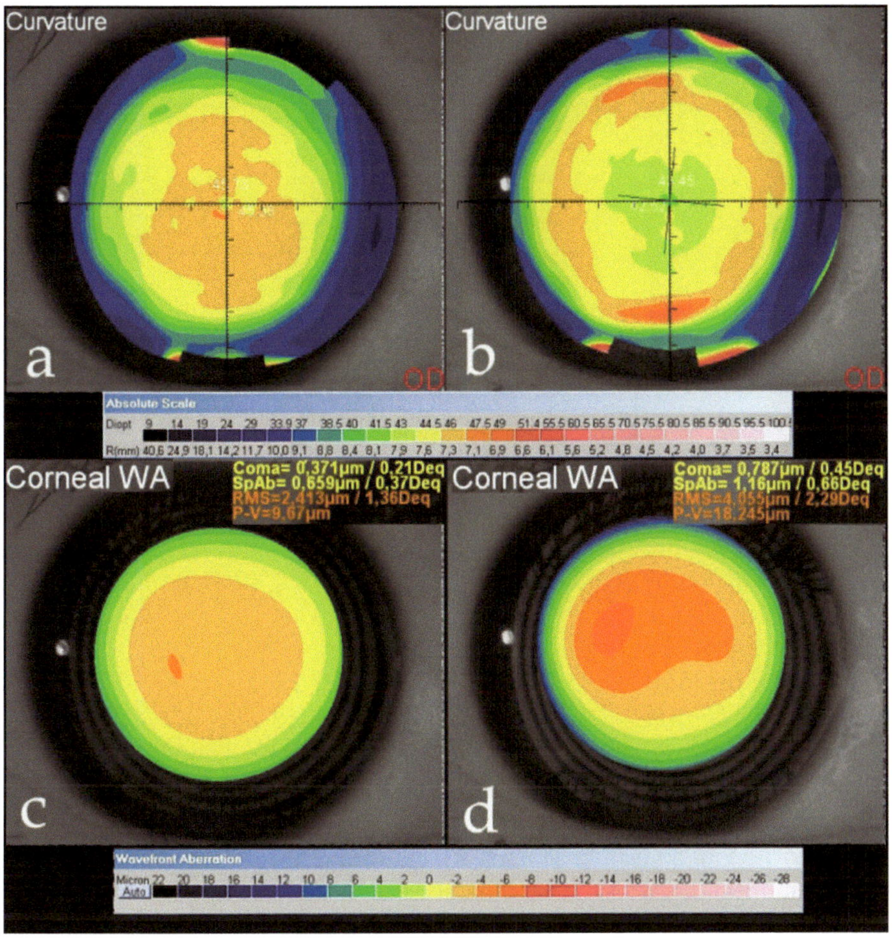

Figure 3-16. Preoperative (A and C) and 1-year postoperative (B and D) tangential and aberrometric topographical images of a patient subjected to an ablation for 3.75 D (myopic) with an optic zone of 6 mm. Note in the images relative to the postoperative period an overall increase in the aberrations, as espressed by the RMS value and in particular the aberrations of 3rd (coma) and 4th (spherical) Zernike's order for a pupil diameter of 7 mm.

the ablation of the meridian of greatest curvature only, and the flatter orthogonal meridian does not change its curvature because it has not been ablated in a homogeneous manner. In this way, the meridian of greatest curvature is flattened but the flatter one is not modified. The oblique meridians are treated in the same way as the main meridian. The imperfect transition also creates a surface with an irregular shape, characterized by evident dioptric variations. In applying the treatment to a single meridian, a multifocal component is induced to the mid-peripheral cornea that is responsible for higher-order aberrations. In 1998, Vinciguerra and colleagues developed an ablation model for the correction of the astigmatic aberrations called *"cross-cylinder ablation."*[101] The technique involved the correction of half of the cylinder along the meridian of greatest curvature and the other half on the flattest meridian. These treatments are joined by the correction of the entire spherical equivalence of the refractive defect. In this way, it is possible to minimize the post-ablation dioptric gradients, with obvious advantages for the quality of vision and the stability and the transparency of the corneal surface. The transition between the treated and untreated portions of cornea becomes more gradual, and some tissue is saved from ablation as the correction of the cylinder is distributed over a large corneal surface (Figure 3-17).

The bitoric ablation, a successive algorithm introduced for the correction of the spherical-cylindrical defect, was described by Chayet and colleagues.[102] This ablation technique is more efficacious in simple and mixed myopic astigmatism. The treatment involves curving the meridian of least curvature and always converting the refractive defect into positive cylinder. For example, +2.00 -4.00 x 180° becomes -2.00 +4.00 x 90° and flattening the meridian of greatest curvature with a myopic ablation, according to the following formula:

$$C_{myo} = \frac{| S + C |}{1.33}$$

$$C_{hyp} = | C | - C_{myo}$$

where the value of C_{myo} (the machine's myopic cylinder setting) is equal to the absolute value of the sum of the preoperative spherical component plus the cylinder divided by 1.33. The value C_{hyp} (the machine's hyperopic cylinder setting) is equal to the absolute value of the negative cylinder.

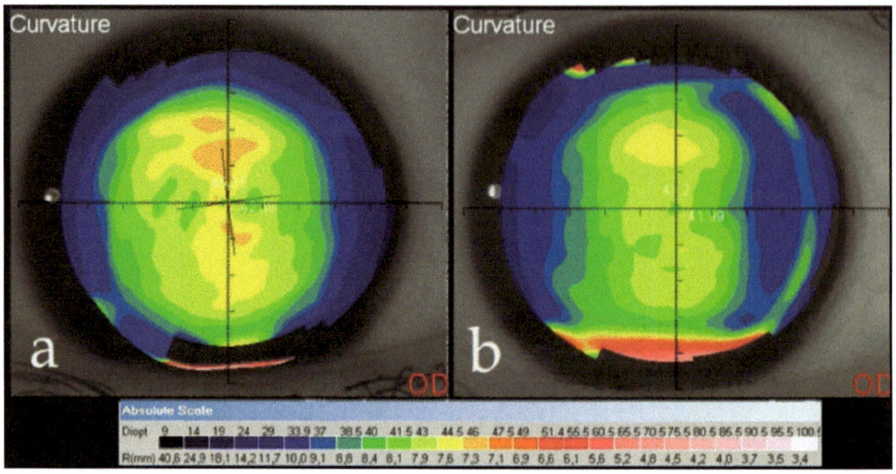

Figure 3-17. Surface ablation performed using the technique of cross-over cylinders for the treatment of mixed astigmatism. (A) The preoperative tangential map. (B) The postoperative situation 1-year after surgery. Note the distribution of treatment on both of the main meridians of the corneal surface.

The ideal pure cylinder corneal ablation should simply reduce the elevation of the corneal plane, maintaining the spherical curvature. As shown in Figure 3-18, the depth of the real and ideal ablation, at the edge of the ablated zone, is zero. The depth of the ideal ablation is increased, but the curvature of the central portion of the cornea is the same as the real ablation. The greater ablation depth "forces" the peripheral portion to be flatter than how it actually results in the real ablation. In other words, the paraxial portion of the ablated corneas with two profiles, real and ideal, have the same curvature. The difference between the two models lies in the peripheral portion, in the transition between the ablated and the non-ablated areas. The ideal aspherical algorithm leads to a lesser curvature in the transition zone with respect to the current ablation models. In theory, this "flattening" of the transition zone will not increase the spherical aberration of the corneal surface. The relative disadvantage is the greater quantity of tissue for ablation required by this ablation model.[103] Nevertheless, the ablation aims to respect the cornea's physiological prolate shape.

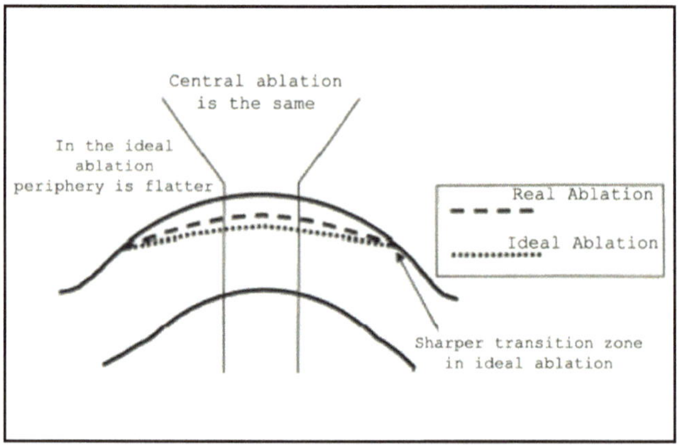

Figure 3-18. Diagram showing the differences between the current real ablation and the ideal aspherical.

Customized Corneal Ablation

A customized ablation has the objective of optimizing the ocular optical system through aspherical and asymmetric algorithms based on the anatomy and on the optical properties of the individual patient's eye. The anatomical factors must take into account the diameter and corneal thicknesses, the depth of the anterior chamber, the pupil diameter under photopic and scotopic conditions, and the dimensions of the crystalline lens. The ocular optic properties are measured as shown, through corneal topography, autorefractometry, ocular aberrometry, and pupillometry. Customized ablation procedures necessitate accurate instruments for the description of corneal morphology, the structure of the ocular optic, and the reshaping of the corneal surface. A system that wishes to support the procedure of customized ablation must be fitted with corneal topography, an ocular wavefront detector, a small spot (≤1 mm) scanning laser, and a valid active system eye-tracker. Corneal topography measures the shape of the corneal surface, not the optical power. The basic measurements of the dimensions and shape of the cornea are as follows:

- The curvature represented by the tangential topographic map.
- The inclination (or slope) of the axial map.
- The height and relative elevation represented by the altitudinal map.

These measurements are correlated but different to each other. The tangential map measures the

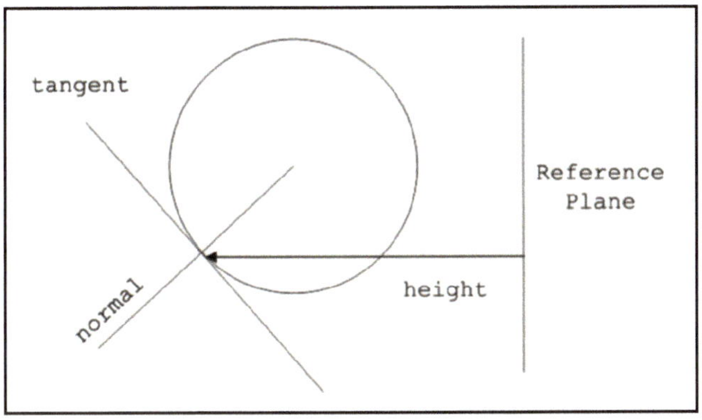

Figure 3-19. The diagram illustrates the geometric constructions required to determine the height and the curvature of a point P of a prolate surface (such as the anterior cornea). The normal situation is the perpendicular local to the surface and passes through the local center of curvature. The inclination refers to the orientation of the tangent through P.

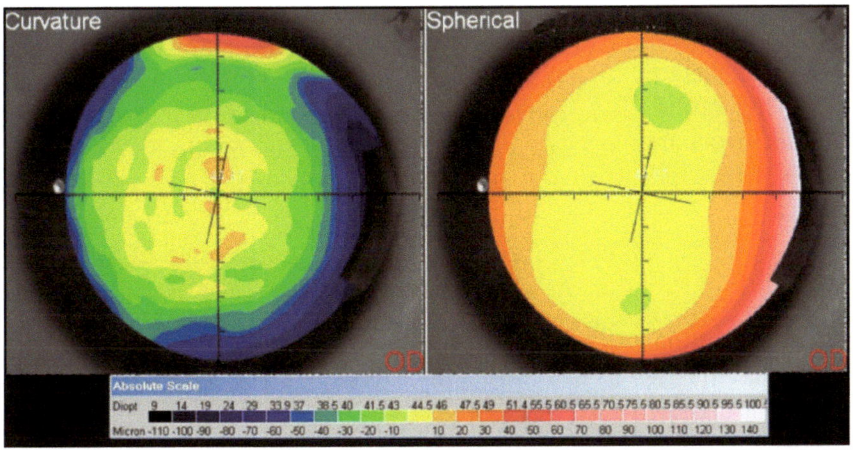

Figure 3-20. Representation of the altitude is performed by subtracting from the profile of the cornea under examination a sphere tangential to the corneal apex. The observation of the altitude maps is espressed in microns. The parts in yellow express the differences close to zero and show the position where the reference spherical surface and the corneal surface coincide. The points where the cornea is above the reference spherical surface are shown in warm colors tending towards red; the points where the cornea lies below the reference surface are shown in colder colors such as greens and blues.

curvature of the cornea and is inversely proportional to the radius of curvature. The inclination measures the angle between the tangent line at a specific point and the normal corneal apex. The height measures the distance between a specific point on the cornea and a plane tangent to the corneal apex; the relative elevation measures the distance between a specific cornea point and a given curved reference surface of known radius (Figure 3-19). On its own, corneal topography cannot define the ideal structure of the anterior cornea, neither can the ideal reference surface for the cornea of the individual patient be calculated on the basis of the topographical measurements alone.

Elevations maps supplied by corneal topography are more appropriate information to guide a customized ablation (Figure 3-20). An accurate system of corneal topography must be able to measure the differences in elevation of the surfaces with a resolution better than 1 μm to be of use in the customized ablation. The common systems of topography based on placido's disk, which exploit the *arc-step* algorithm, can detect variations in elevation of the corneal surface of up to 0.7 μm (which corresponds to a modification of the wavefront of 0.48 wave). These systems provide the best resolution available at present.[104]

The aberrometers provide information on the total and corneal ocular optic properties. The correlation of the figures supplied by the detection systems for the ocular and corneal wavefronts are the critical factor in the individual patient's quest for perfect vision. Aberrations from the corneal surface and the lens generally tend to counterbalance each other, particularly in younger patients. Modifications to the aberrometric maps of the corneal surface must take the intraocular optical aberrations into account. The "aberration-free" corneal ablation must correspond to the following equation:

$$W(x, y)\ corneal = W(x,y)\ ocular - W(x,y)\ intraocular$$

This formula relies on the understanding that not all of the aberrations from the corneal surface are corrected to avoid upsetting the equilibrium with the intraocular aberrations.

At the time of writing, no laser device exists that can interface the aberrometry of the first corneal surface and the ocular aberrometry. The commercially available systems are guided by topography *(topo-link)* or aberrometry *(wavefront-guided).*

The basic ablation formula under topo-link can be expressed through the following:

$$A(x, y) = C - (T [x, y] - T_{target} [x, y])$$

where A(x, y) is the ablation pattern, T (x,y) is the real altitude corneal topography, T_{target} (x, y) is the ideal topography desired, and C is the smallest depth constant to maintain A(x, y) above negative values at any point. The ablation depth A(x, y) cannot be allowed to reach negative values because an ablation cannot add tissue to the cornea. C is equal to the maximum value of ($T[x, y] - T_{target}[x, y]$) within the optic zone. In theory, $T_{target}(x, y)$ should be a parabolic surface with a refractive power suitable for achieving emmetropia or other refractive targets. Wavefront errors are described in polar coordinates by W (r, Θ), where n = 1.3771 is the refractive index of the cornea.

$$Z_{abl}(r, \theta) = \frac{w(r, \theta)}{N - 1}$$

There are some essential features of this equation. First, the wavefront error must be measured accurately on the corneal front (the shape of the wavefront changes as it propagates through space). Second, when a luminous ray passes through a cornea that has not been ablated, it follows a specific course through the other surfaces of the eye. The ablation profile has also been designed to compensate for the aberrations introduced by the posterior corneal surface and the lens.

Following the ablation, the beam follows a slightly different pathway, and the aberrating components of the posterior surface of the cornea and the lens will be slightly different from the situation prior to the treatment. The equation described above is an expression of the fact that the ablation model compensates the aberrations of a given light beam along its pathway inside the eye, even if this beam follows a slightly different pathway following ablation.

Under experimental conditions, it has been shown that the ideal beam for the customized ablation must be Gaussian. A Gaussian beam will allow an extremely uniform superimposition of the ablation profile.[105] The spot dimensions must correspond to the resolution of the aberrations to be treated. It has been calculated that a spot of diameter less than 1 mm allows the correction of aberrations superior to Zernike's fourth order. Finally, the scanning of the spot should be nonsequential with regards to the pulse position (two successive pulses should not be adjacent) to avoid any increase in temperature of the corneal stroma. On the other hand, a reduction in the spot diameter will lead to an increase in the sensitivity to errors associated with the laser position. For a customized ablation, it is essential that every spot be localized accurately on the corneal plane. The key to a result close to the desired value is to achieve real-time alignment between the laser and the reference coordinate system: the eye-tracking systems were developed for this purpose.[106]

When the patient is fixating the target light, frequent saccadic eye movements are recorded. Their main characteristics are the randomness and the rapid frequency (approximately five per second). Consequently, an accurate correction system necessitates an efficacious eye-tracker. The fixation saccadic eye movements cover a distance of 1° to 10° (0.1 to 0.2 mm), at a frequency of 100°/sec to 800°/sec (22 to 170 mm/sec). In order to adequately follow the saccadic movements during fixation, a wide-band (100-Hz) eye-tracker is essential. The final step of integration of the ablation profile on the basis of the wavefront necessitates understanding of the variables associated with the corneal response to photoablation, and these include the epithelial-stromal remodeling and the corneal biomechanical response.

Clinical Results of Customized Ablations

The preparation procedures for a patient undergoing a customized treatment are basically the same as the standard procedure from the surgical perspective. The difference between the treatment lies with the fact that the eye's topographical or aberrometric parameters are recorded and transferred to the laser system in order to personalize the ablation profile. During the preoperative evaluation, it is essential to understand the causes of blurred vision through an accurate topographical or aberrometric examination. The objective of customized refractive surgery is to improve the patient's current visual performance; consequently, it is essential that the patient understand the potential results of the treatment compared to his or her real expectations. The first personalized treatments were performed on corneas that had already been treated with radial keratotomy,[107] keratoplasty, or a previous photorefractive surgery to minimize the effects of astigmatism or higher-order aberrations. At a later stage, the customized treatment was extended to include healthy eyes to improve the quality of the patient's natural sight under every condition of

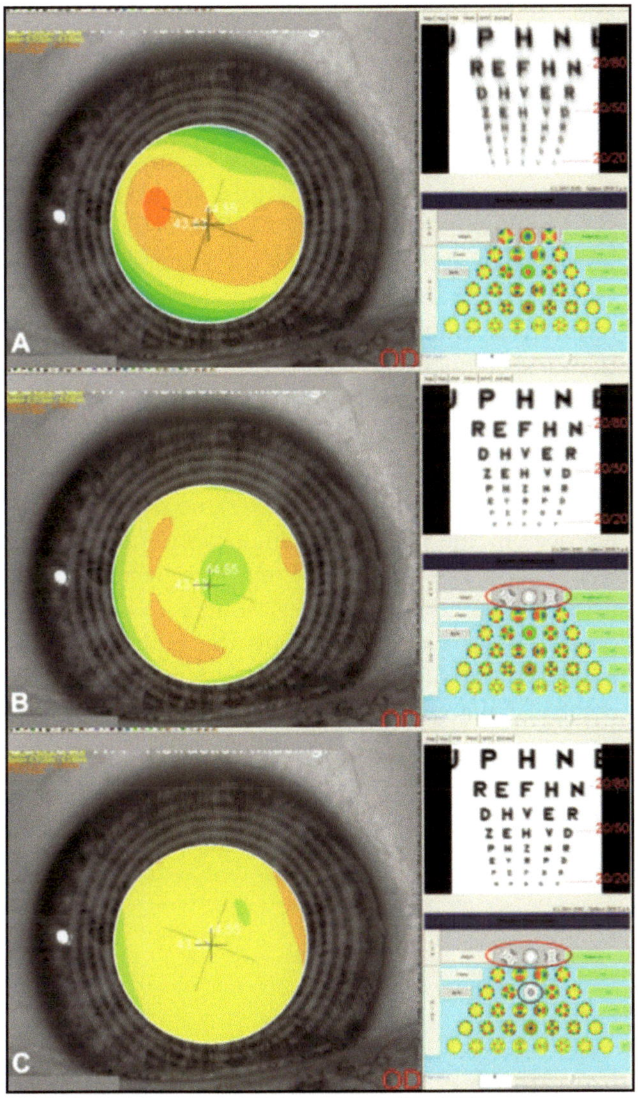

Figure 3-21. Preoperative corneal aberrometry with simulation of the visual acuity on the Ottotipo LogMAR (the last line corresponds to 10/10) for a pupil diameter of 6 mm. (A) The current visual acuity of the patient with a refractive defect of -2.50 sph = -0.50 cyl @ 180°. (B) The visual acuity following the correction of defocus and astigmatism. (C) The visual acuity following the correction of the spherical aberration. It is clear how the quality of vision improves under scotopic conditions following the correction of high-order aberrations.

lighting, particularly for eyes with a high preoperative RMS of higher-order aberrations. It is clear that the preoperative discussion with the patient depends on the type of treatment or enhancement planned. In the case of previously operated patients with residual myopic or hyperopic defocus or elevated or irregular astigmatism, the focus of the discussion must be the improvement in natural visual acuity and vision quality in daylight and not the elimination of every optical defect in the eye to produce super-vision. The patient must be fully informed of this. It is possible to use the visual simulation functions of the corneal ocular aberrometers; by modifying the value of the high and/or low optic aberrations, it is possible to illustrate the patient's postoperative performance (Figure 3-21). Pseudophakic patients, patients subjected to perforating keratoplasty or following radial keratotomy, treated with a standard PRK procedure with residual refractive or invalidating higher-order aberrations can benefit from the customized topo-link or wavefront-guided treatment.

For healthy patients subjected to a customized refractive surgery treatment, the surgeon should perform a detailed examination of the total RMS of the higher-order aberrations under scotopic conditions. This will supply the best possible operating indications. Eyes with total higher-order RMS superior to 0.8 μm for pupil diameters that are equal to or less than 6 mm can benefit from customized treatment. Alternately, similar results can be achieved with an aspherical treatment. In fact, the international literature reports that the results achieved with the topo-link treatments performed with the current laser systems do not differ greatly from the wavefront-guided treatments in terms of less induction of optical aberrations or a reduction in contrast sensitivity.

The exact difference in the shape of the personalized ablation profile of the individual laser system is not a known entity. All of the surgical platforms follow the same principles, once the eye's topographical and/or aberrometric information has been obtained, it is uploaded into the laser system, which then designs the treatment.

The de-epithelialization procedure of the cornea follows the same principles as those applied to the standard PRK. The eye-tracker is activated, and the ablation process begins.

Medication of the eye subjected to a customized surface surgical procedure is identical to the standard procedure. The patient will be given exactly the same advice to follow postoperatively (detailed information in the informed consent form).

During the past 5 years, numerous articles have been published on the clinical refractive and aberrometric results of customized surface treatments. The more important results from each of the currently available laser systems are summarized below.

In a prospective clinical trial[108] with the Technolas 217Z (Bausch + Lomb) excimer laser used for the treatment of moderate myopia in a group of 56 patients, the customized treatment induced a smaller quantity of coma with respect to the standard PlanoScan treatment. In a prospective study[109] of 28 patients with a mean spherical refractive defect of approximately -5 D and a cylindrical defect of approximately 1 D, half of whom were subjected to customized PRK and the other half subjected to the standard PRK treatment with the Technolas 217Z laser system, no significant differences in the increase of higher-order aberrations were observed within the optic zone nor in the reduction of the contrast sensitivity at approximately 9 months from surgery.

In a prospective study[110] of 56 patients, subjected at random to PRK with an aspherical profile or customized PRK using the Wavelight Eye Q (Alcon Laboratories, Fort Worth, TX) laser system, no significant differences were measured in the increase of higher-order aberrations between the two treatments performed for the correction of moderate myopia (up to -6 D) and astigmatism of up to 2.5 D. In a recent prospective study,[111] two groups of patients were randomized for the customized topo-link treatment (Allegretto Topolyzer) or the wavefront-guided treatment (Allegretto Wave) using the WaveLight system for the correction of moderate myopia. The results after 6 months of follow-up showed no significant difference in the increase of higher-order optical aberrations or in the reduction of contrast sensitivity between the two types of treatment.

In another prospective study,[112] 126 myopic patients were subjected, respectively, to a standard ablation (48 eyes) with the MEL 70G (Asclepion Meditec) laser system and to a customized treatment (78 eyes) with the WASCA system. The customized treatment induced a lower quantity of higher-order aberrations—specifically, coma and spherical aberrations.

In a retrospective study that examined 226 myopic patients treated with the NAVEX (Nidek) system using the topo-link (CATz, 158 eyes) or a wavefront-guided system (OPDCAT, 68 eyes), no significant differences in the quantity of higher-order aberrations were found at 1-year follow-up. In another study[113] using the same NAVEX laser source, the CATz and OPDCAT were compared with the aspherical treatment (OATz) in a group of 1459 myopic eyes. The results of the study were similar for all of the ablation profiles, even if the topo-link treatment allowed greater predictability of the results up to 1 year after surgery.

Conclusions

Where the surgeon is concerned, scientific theories behind the various procedures should require the indispensable principle to optimize the results. In corneal refractive surgery, knowledge of the healing processes, the optical properties of the virgin corneal surface, the structure of the corneal tissue, the ablation models, and the instruments in use are all essential to provide the patient the best results possible and an improvement in visual performance.

In-depth knowledge of the epithelial-stromal remodeling process may suggest new opportunities to modulate the physiopathological response of the cornea and to maintain the optic properties of the corneal tissue, namely transparency and asphericity.

At the time of writing, the only pharmacological agents widely used to control the postoperative biological response of the cornea are topical corticosteroids or mitomycin C. They act by inhibiting the activated keratocytes. However, there is considerable controversial data available on the indiscriminate use of corticosteroids following any surgical operation with the excimer laser.[114,115] The biophysical response of corneal tissue to a surgical procedure that aims to modify the optical properties by intervening on the morphological profile of the tissue itself is the main variable of refractive surgery with excimer laser. Optimizing the results of refractive surgery necessitates the solution of several variables, including the following:

1. The differences of the corneal optics and biomechanics between individuals, such as modifications of the eye's aberrometric map (of the cornea or of the intraocular optical surfaces) as the patient ages, the modifications of the pupil diameter under conditions of different illumination and accommodation, the properties of the lacrimal film due to frequent alterations in the healthy population, such as dry eye and blepharitis, the variations of the biomechanical properties, and the thickness of the various corneal quadrants.
2. The complex and undefined process of epithelial and stromal healing.
3. The technological limits, which may be minimal, such as the alignment and the position of the eye during the phases of topographical and aberrometric measurement and during the surgical procedure and the ablation accuracy of the laser system.
4. Surgeon's errors including inaccuracies in the preoperative measurements, the environmental characteristics of the operating room, and the dryness or the excessive hydration of the ocular surface during surgery.[116]

Despite the technical limitations, it is an undeniable fact that many patients today enjoy extremely satisfactory natural visual quality. Personalized vision

Buratto L, Slade S, Serrao S, Lombardo M. *PRK: The Past, Present, and Future of Surface Ablation. (pp. 49-50).*

correction is the most advanced and valid model for providing excellent visual performance to the majority of patients. The personalized correction of the ocular optical aberrations requires the precise measurement of the error of the wavefront and accurate systems of surgical correction. If the cornea was a stiff material and if its mechanical properties did not change with time, this model of customized ablation would be perfect for the correction of monochromatic aberrations of the eye. The objective of the customized ablation is to optimize the visual performance; the strategy used is to minimize the ocular optical aberrations. The introduction of variables from the cornea's postoperative biophysical response to the ablation algorithm would be ideal.

To optimize the patient's vision quality, the surgeon must not underestimate the role of the orthoptic condition in each subject and, in particular, the functional and sensory equilibriums, which may be disturbed by the treatment of the optical aberrations in one or both eyes. The same lack of perfect orthophoria can introduce lower-order aberrations such as *tilt,* despite the hypothetical correction of all of the ocular aberrations. In a significant number of patients, particularly those with asymmetrical and/or high refractive defects, an accurate orthoptic evaluation prior to surgery is indispensable in order to exclude the possible appearance of oculo-motory decompensation or evident diplopia.[117]

One extremely interesting area that attempts to "correct" the ablation is *real-time topography.* At the time of writing, the laser industries are studying means of how to achieve the real-time image of the changes in the shape of the cornea during treatment. Such a device would provide true potential for modifying the plan of the correction procedure in real time in relation to the individualized biomechanical response, in order to optimize the end result. In conclusion, laser refractive surgery today aims not only to eliminate traditional defects of ocular refraction but also to produce an improvement in the visual performance and quality for the individual patient. This surgical approach must take a number of anatomical, functional, and social factors into account, personalizing the choice to provide better quality vision for the individual.

ATTACHMENTS

Attachment 1

INFORMATION DATA SHEET ATTACHED TO THE INFORMED CONSENT FOR THE KERATECTOMY PROCEDURE WITH EXCIMER LASER:

Dear Sir/Madam,

As you are aware, your eyes are affected by a refractive defect: myopia, hyperopia, or astigmatism. Until recently, these sight defects were corrected with spectacles or contact lenses; now, there is a therapeutic alternative with a para-surgical operation using an excimer laser. This letter contains information about the treatment itself, the expected results, and the risks associated with the surgery. All of the technical expressions used in this document will be integrated with a detailed verbal explanatory description.

In the normal eye, the pathway of the light rays is modified by the cornea and the crystalline lens to ensure the rays will converge on the retina. In the myopic eye, because the eye is longer than normal, the rays converge in front of the retina. In the hyperopic eye, which is shorter than a normal eye, the rays will converge behind the retina. The astigmatic eye is affected by anomalies in the corneal curvature. If the desire to avoid wearing corrective lenses for aesthetic reasons is excluded, refractive surgery will bring maximum advantage when the ocular and environmental parameters prevent the patient from maximizing his or her visual capacity. This is more evident when there are severe visual defects that bind the patient to the use of corrective lenses, when there are major differences in refraction between one eye and the other, particularly when the patient is intolerant to contact lenses, and when the patient's employment places him or her at a disadvantage if he or she is obliged to use corrective lenses.

Careful patient selection by the doctor, the specific clinical characteristics, and in-depth investigation into the reasons why the patient has opted for the operation are absolutely essential components of the preoperative procedures. This type of surgery is irreversible, complications may arise, and secondary modifications may be necessary. Other symptoms include persistence or appearance of undesired residual refractive defects, all problems that are common to ocular surgery.

It should also be emphasized that every refractive surgery, irrespective of the technique used, is oriented to resolving the defects of refraction alone and will

Buratto L, Slade S, Serrao S, Lombardo M. *PRK: The Past, Present, and Future of Surface Ablation. (pp. 51-56).*

not modify other pathologies that are associated with the vision defect. For example, a patient affected by myopia with retinal alterations that compromise the visual function cannot expect to resolve this problem simply by undergoing refractive surgery. This type of surgery cannot protect the patient against any successive retinal complications. The operation aims to reduce the power of the lenses used or, in the most successful cases, can eliminate them completely with a reduction in the discomfort and distortions that accompany them.

So, to avoid errors and misunderstandings regarding the scheduled surgical program and the results achievable, the doctor must give the patient a detailed explanation of every aspect of the procedure. In this way, the patient will sign the consent form fully convinced of the benefits and risks associated with procedure he or she is undertaking. A patient who demands natural 10/10 vision should be excluded from surgery, as minimum residual refractive defects may persist. These depend on the biological variables of each individual and are factors that cannot be easily predicted.

It is also unlikely that following surgery, an amblyopic patient (with a lazy eye) will perceive any improvement in his or her visual acuity. Moreover, the operation does not prevent the physiological development of presbyopia, and in particular, in patients with early manifestations of the disorder, the complete elimination of the myopic effect will necessitate correction for near vision.

According to your eye doctor, you could benefit from corneal remodeling with an excimer laser. In those cases where surgery is required to satisfy the conditions of a job application (a career with the military, pilot's license, etc), the patient must obtain the information relative to the visual characteristics requested in the job description and the legitimacy of the surgical operation in relation to the type of employment.

Prior to surgery, the use of contact lenses must be suspended some days prior to treatment (according to the surgeon's instructions). The surgeon will also give the patient the necessary advice regarding his or her ocular or medical therapies.

It is a legal requirement to read and sign the informed consent form if surgery is to occur.

Technique

The excimer laser is a modern instrument that can remove microscopic fragments of corneal tissue from the surface (PRK technique) or in the intermediate layer (LASIK technique). It does this with a laser light beam in the UV spectrum. The tissue is removed with extraordinary precision, which is impossible by manual techniques, just 0.25 μm (one-thousandth of a millimeter) for every pulse emitted. The accuracy of the result cannot be achieved with any other instrument. In particular, the accuracy of this instrument is exploited to remodel the central corneal curvature. In this way, it is possible to eliminate or reduce the refractive defects: myopia, hyperopia, and astigmatism (though the treatment success for the latter two is much lower).

Day of Surgery

It is preferable, though not indispensable, to be accompanied to the surgical center. The eye may be bandaged after treatment (and this may cause problems with driving). Ladies must not wear make-up or perfume (the alcohol vapors from the products can interfere with the laser beam). The patient must also bring the results of the preliminary tests, his or her medical record, and this letter with him or her to the surgical center on the day of surgery.

The PRK technique proceeds as follows:

1. The surgeon instills a few drops of anesthetic onto the surface of the eye.
2. The patient is positioned on the surgical bed beneath the laser machine;
3. The surgeon applies a small eyelid speculum.
4. A portion of the thin surface membrane of the cornea is removed (epithelium).
5. The optic center of the eye is "memorized" by the eye-tracker by asking the patient to fixate on a small red luminous target spot.
6. The laser treatment begins.
7. After treatment, the surgeon medicates the eye with eye drops and applies a therapeutic contact lens; he or she may also ask the patient to wear a protective shell or a patch.

The operation is performed in the Day Hospital or outpatient center. Removal of the epithelium lasts approximately 2 minutes and the laser treatment an additional 2 minutes.

The operation is typically painless, although the patient may have some discomfort caused by the eyelid speculum.

In some suitable cases, the ophthalmic surgeon may opt for LASIK, a variation of the above technique. In this case, the excimer laser treatment is not performed on the surface of the cornea, but in the intermediate layers. For this technique to be used, prior to treatment with the excimer laser, the surgeon must perform a small lamellar incision with a mechanical instrument such as a microkeratome or a femtosecond laser platform.

This surgical technique can be compared to opening a book (the action involved in creating the corneal lamella or flap, using a microkeratome or the femtosecond laser), the removal of some pages inside the cover (laser action), and closing the book (repositioning the lamellae). In some cases, temporary sutures may be necessary at the end of surgery. If the surgeon decides that the lamellar cut is poor quality, the flap should be replaced, and surgery should be deferred to a later date, to be decided by the surgeon. All eye surgeons agree with this line of thinking.

There is no major difference in the type of anesthesia used (both techniques are performed under local anesthesia with eye drops), and there is no difference in the duration of the two operations. During surgery, it is possible that patients' vision is temporarily blurred. This is normal and should not be a cause for worry. Patient cooperation is an essential factor in achieving an excellent result, as the patient must follow all of the instructions given to him or her by the surgeon before and during surgery. At the end of the procedure, the surgeon will prescribe drug therapy of eye drops and tablets that must be followed carefully during the postoperative period.

Postoperative Course

The patient must medicate his or her eye with the prescribed drops starting on the day of surgery. In the initial 24 to 48 hours following the PRK operation, the patient may feel discomfort and/or pain of varying intensity in his or her eye. Normally, the treatment prescribed can control this pain and keep it at acceptable levels. The bandages or patches can usually be removed from the eye after 48 to 72 hours. The postoperative course following LASIK is generally pain-free. The patient may perceive the sensation of a foreign body in the eye or a burning sensation. The bandages are removed from the eye soon after surgery; however, the patient must not rub or manipulate the eyelid in any way for at least 1 month.

The doctor will re-call the patient for control visits at intervals after surgery. These controls are essential and obligatory to allow the surgeon to check the progression of the operated eye. Failure to follow the postoperative therapy and to attend the specialist controls may affect the final refractive result and lead to complications. It is therefore of fundamental importance to carefully follow the surgeon's prescriptions, which are devised to facilitate the healing processes and produce a more satisfactory result.

Following surgery, the patient is permitted to read, write, and watch television. For approximately 1 month after surgery, the patient should avoid any sporting activities that involve physical contact, driving a motorcycle, applying makeup, and frequenting saunas and swimming pools. Once the post operative controls have terminated, the patient should be checked on an annual basis. He or she should inform his or her eye doctor (if different from the doctor who performed the surgery) that he or she was subjected to excimer laser treatment, as special attention must be taken by the doctor when ocular pressure is measured.

Visual Recovery

Visual recovery will be progressive, over the first few weeks following surgery, and transitional hyperopia of variable duration may appear (it may last 1 or 2 months). This may cause problems with near vision and focus, which will make reading difficult. Moreover, the different refraction between the two eyes, which will be apparent following the operation on the first eye, can provoke visual discomfort and a feeling of disorientation. During this period, there are no particular restrictions in terms of professional activities or social commitments. Patients should use their common sense as their vision is still imperfect. Complete visual recovery (that is, achievement of the preset objectives) is reached after a certain period of time (from between 1 and 6 months, depending on the entity of the defect corrected).

Refractive Results

The surgical treatment with the latest-generation excimer laser is the most precise method available today for the correction of myopia, hyperopia, and astigmatism. This instrument with almost absolute precision treats the visual defects. Nevertheless, events beyond the surgeon's control (in terms of his technique and the precision of the laser) can affect the healing process and the visual outcome. As a result, an accurate prediction of the achievable optic correction is not possible.

Modest differences from the expected result (hypo- or hypercorrection within ±0.75 D) are possible and cannot be defined as unsuccessful surgery. The initial result may regress with time; however, in the majority of cases, the improvement in vision will usually be sufficient to allow the patient to eliminate spectacles or contact lenses. In some cases (<5%), additional correction with spectacles or contact lenses may be necessary. Enhancement treatments may be recommended by the surgeon to reduce residual refractive or scar-based defects.

Complications

Complications are a risk with any surgical procedure. Zero-risk operations do not exist now and are unlikely to exist in the future.

Your eye surgeon is therefore unable to guarantee the absolute success of the surgery.

In addition to the common surgical complications (infections, instrument malfunction, etc), treatment with the excimer laser is associated with the following rare complications:

a) Transitory corneal opacities may appear during the healing process. Initially, this opacity may cause minor reductions in the visual efficiency; however, it will normally regress within 6 months.

b) Irregularities of the corneal surface may lead to a temporary and minor reduction in visual acuity. These will also tend to regress over time.

c) Irregularities of the corneal healing, which will affect the corneal surface and produce distorted images, create ghost images or lead to a permanent reduction in the maximum visual acuity.

d) Sometimes, in the initial postoperative period, the patient may perceive halos around light sources and glare, particularly at night. This phenomenon is well tolerated and will generally regress completely within a few months and after the treatment has been performed on both eyes.

e) Other rare complications include corneal ulcers, non-specific widespread interstitial keratitis, corneal melting, a loss of corneal endothelial cells, progressive thinning of the cornea, formation of or an increase in the number of mobile bodies, retinal hemorrhage, and detachment of the retina.

f) In refractive surgery, as for any other form of ocular surgery, the complications can be serious (for example, when infections do not respond to antibiotic and/or steroid therapies) and may lead to the loss of vision or, in extreme case, complete loss of the eye. These complications are so exceptional that it is impossible to calculate the frequency of their occurrence.

g) As the excimer laser treatment is a fairly recent development, it is possible that other complications exist that have still not been reported. The results of long-term studies may reveal additional risks. The patient should therefore be checked routinely to evaluate the condition of his or her eyes. The LASIK technique is also associated with specific complications caused by instrument malfunction when cutting the lamella (the microkeratome or the femtosecond laser) with consequent damage to the flap; in some rare cases, an irregular cut can lead to blurred or distorted vision. As mentioned earlier, in this case, the surgeon may decide to defer surgery to a later date. In order to prevent these unexpected events, prior to every operation, the surgeon and his or her technicians should perform the necessary electro-mechanical controls to ensure the good function of the instruments.

Your eye surgeon will be happy to answer any questions you have.

Your doctor is legally required to prove that he or she has provided the necessary information regarding the surgery to the patient. You are therefore asked to sign this document and the informed consent form.

I hereby declare that I have read and understood the above document.

Date: ______________________________

For acceptance (patient's legible signature)

____

Attachment 2

Informed Consent

I, the undersigned, ____________________, date of birth ______________, place of birth ______________, resident in ________________, with this, a full, free-willed and unconditional expression of my wishes,

Declare

that I am in full possession of all my mental faculties and I wish to undergo the operation of refractive surgery by excimer laser. I have been given a full and comprehensive explanation of the characteristics of the operation and have carefully examined all of the information given to me and summarized in a specific memorandum that I have signed (as read, understood, and accepted, with said document attached to this informed consent). I am fully aware of the benefits and generic and specific risks associated with the operation.

I also state that I am aware I may be affected by:

1. Glare and/or photophobia, which may appear in the initial postoperative phases;
2. Generic and specific complications as a result of the operation;
3. The consequences of negligence on my part regarding the postoperative therapeutic and behavioral practices, prescribed to me by the surgeon immediately after surgery and during the postoperative control visits. I accept that I must follow the scheduled therapy precisely.

The benefits aim for the total elimination of corrective lenses or a reduction in their power. However, I accept that, under specific conditions, the use of corrective lenses may still be necessary.

I declare that I was given the opportunity to ask my surgeon and his or her staff any questions or about any doubts I had regarding this operation and that I was given precise, clear, and detailed answers.

I also declare that I was informed that there are events, which are beyond the control of the surgeon's hands and the precision of the laser, that may affect the healing process and consequently the outcome of surgery. As a result, I am aware that it is impossible to formulate an absolute prediction regarding the optic correction achievable. Presuming the surgeon's professional diligence, I relieve him or her of all levels of civil responsibility associated with a partial or total lack of the result.

I am aware that my visual acuity prior to surgery is:

R ______/______ natural; _______/_______
with ________ sph ________ cyl axis ________

L ______/______ natural; _______/_______
with ________ sph ________ cyl axis ________

As was clearly explained to me, the visual capacity depends on the overall conditions of my sight organs. The photoablative treatment will at least maintain the maximum preoperative visual acuity with optical correction or, in the more successful cases, with no need for correction.

Nevertheless, I am fully aware that the photorefractive treatment cannot prevent any modifications or deteriorations of the visual acuity caused by any subsequent modification of the refractive defect or damage caused by any other pathology.

I declare that I am fully aware of the option of enhancement treatments should they prove necessary. These will be performed at the discretion of the surgeon who will intervene in the attempt to reduce any residual refractive defects or distortions caused by healing.

Operation: Right Eye <> PRK <> LASIK <>
Date: ____
Legible signature:
Operation: Left Eye <> PRK <> LASIK <>
Date: ____
Legible Signature:
____

I declare that I have read and understood all of the information given to me. I also declare that all the blank spaces were filled prior to me signing the forms.

Dr. ____________________________________ will be responsible for the medical-surgical treatment.

References

1. Liang J, Williams DR. Aberrations and retinal image quality of the normal human eye. *J Opt Soc Am Assoc.* 1997;14:2873-2883.
2. Applegate RA. Limits to vision: can we do better than nature? *J Refract Surg.* 2000;16:S547-S551.
3. Williams D, Yoon GY, Porter J, Guirao A, Hofer H. Visual benefit of correcting higher order aberrations of the eye. *J Refract Surg.* 2000;16:S554-S559.
4. Thibos LN. The prospects for perfect vision. *J Refract Surg.* 2000;16:S540-S546.
5. Campbell FW, Green DG. Optical and retinal factors affecting visual resolution. *J Physiol.* 1965;181:576-593.
6. Anhalt GJ, Jampel HD. Bullous autoantibodies are markers of corneal epithelial hemidesmosomes. *Invest Ophthalmol Vis Sci.* 1987;28:903-907.
7. Renard G, Montanez-Mendoza M, Savoldelli M, Pouliquen Y. Scanning microscopy study of the corneal epithelium. Relation of various aspects to the lacrimal film. *J Fr Ophtalmol.* 1983;6:697-705.
8. Tsilimbaris MK, Lesnieswska E, Lydataki S, Le Grimellec C, Goudonnet JP, Pallikaris IG. The use of atomic force microscopy for the observation of corneal epithelium surface. *Invest Ophthalmol Vis Sci.* 2000;41:680-686.
9. Borcherding MS, Blacik LJ. Proteoglycans and collagen fibre organization in human corneoscleral tissue. *Exp Eye Res.* 1975;21:59-70.
10. Meek KM, Fullwood NJ. Corneal and scleral collagens—a microscopist's perspective. *Micron.* 2001;32:261-272.
11. Meller D, Peters K, Meller K. Human cornea and sclera studied by atomic force microscopy. *Cell Tissue Res.* 1997;288:111-118.
12. Maurice DM. The structure and transparency of the corneal stroma. *J Physiol.* 1957;136:263-286.
13. Sandler SS. Direct three-dimensional reconstruction of a corneal stromal lamella from electron micrographs. *J Theoret Biol.* 1974;48:207-213.
14. Maurice DM. The transparency of the corneal stroma. *Vision Res.* 1970;10:107-108.
15. Muller LJ, Pels E, Vrensen GF. The specific architecture of the anterior stroma accounts for maintenance of corneal curvature. *Br J Ophthalmol.* 2001;85:437-443.
16. Versura P, Bovincini F. Scanning electron microscopy of normal human cornea and conjunctiva in normal and pathological conditions. *Scanning Electron Microsc.* 1985;4:1695-1708.
17. Jones MA, Manfurt CF. Sympathetic stimulation of corneal epithelial proliferation in wounded and nonwounded rat eyes. *Invest Ophthalmol Vis Sci.* 1996;37:2535-2547.
18. Tutt R, Bradley A, Begley C, Thibos LN. Optical and visual impact of tear break-up in human eyes. *Invest Ophthalmol Vis Sci.* 2000;41:4117-4123.
19. Huang FC, Tseng SH, Shih MH, Chen FK. Effect of artificial tears on corneal surface regularity, contrast sensitivity, and glare disability in dry eyes. *Ophthalmology.* 2002;109:1934-1940.
20. Davanger M, Evenson A. Role of the pericorneal structure in renewal of corneal epithelium. *Nature.* 1971;229:560-561.
21. Daniels JT, Dart JKG, Tuft SJ, Khaw PT. Corneal stem cells in review. *Wound Rep Reg.* 2001;9:483-494.
22. Schofield R. The stem cell system. *Biomed Pharmacother.* 1983;37:375-380.

Buratto L, Slade S, Serrao S, Lombardo M. ***PRK: The Past, Present, and Future of Surface Ablation. (pp. 57-62).***

23. Tseng SC. Regulation and clinical implications of corneal epithelial stem cells. *Mol Biol Rep.* 1996;23:47-58.
24. Wilson SE, Mohan RR, Mohan RR, Ambrosio R Jr, Hong J, Lee J. The corneal wound healing response: cytokine-mediated interaction of the epithelium, stroma, and inflammatory cells. *Prog Retin Eye Res.* 2001;20:625-637.
25. Thoft RA, Friend J. The X, Y, Z hypothesis of corneal epithelial maintenance. *Invest Ophthalmol Vis Sci.* 1983;24:1442-1443.
26. Ren H, Wilson G. The cell shedding rate of the corneal epithelium—a comparison of collection methods. *Curr Eye Res.* 1996;15:1054-1059.
27. Pfister RR. Clinical measures to promote corneal epithelial healing. *Acta Ophthalmol Scand.* 1992;202(suppl):73-83.
28. Mauger TF, Hill RM. Corneal epithelial healing under contact lenses: quantitative analysis in the rabbit. *Acta Ophthalmol Scand.* 1992;70:361-365.
29. Gaffney EA, Maini PK, Sherratt JA, Tuft S. The mathematical modelling of cell kinetics in corneal epithelial wound healing. *J Theor Biol.* 1999;197:15-40.
30. Crosson CE, Klyce SD, Beuerman RW. Epithelial wound closure in the rabbit cornea. A biphasic process. *Invest Ophthalmol Vis Sci.* 1986;27:464-473.
31. Estil S, Kravik K, Haaskjold E, Refsum SB, Bjerkness R, Wilson G. Pilot study on the time course of apoptosis in the regenerating corneal epithelium. *Acta Ophthalmol Scand.* 2002;80:517.
32. Haaskjold E, Refsum SB, Bjerkness R. Circadian variation in the mitotic rate of the corneal epithelium. Cell division and migration are analyzed by a mathematical model. *Virchows Arch B Cell Pathol.* 1989;58:123-127.
33. Estil S, Haaskjold E, Bjerkness R, Refsum SB. A previous abrasion in the contralateral eye influences the cell kinetics during healing of a central corneal abrasion. *Acta Ophthalmol Scand.* 2001;79:389-395.
34. Rask R, Koch JO, Ehlers N. Epithelial healing in the second eye after corneal abrasion. *Acta Ophthalmol Scand.* 1996;74:232-234.
35. Gipson IK, Spurr-Michaud S, Tisdale A, Keough M. Reassembly of the anchoring structure of the corneal epithelium during wound repair in the rabbit. *Invest Ophthalmol Vis Sci.* 1989;30:425-434.
36. Lu L, Reinach PS, Kao WWY. Corneal epithelial wound healing. *Exp Biol Med.* 2001;226:653-664.
37. Weiss RA, Liaw LHL, Berns M, Amoils SP. Scanning electron microscopy comparison of corneal epithelial removal techniques before photorefractive keratectomy. *J Cataract Refract Surg.* 1999;25:1093-1096.
38. Vinciguerra P, Albè E, Camesasca FI, Trazza S, Epstein D. Wavefront- versus topography-guided customized ablations with the NIDEK EC-5000 CX II in surface ablation treatment: refractive and aberrometric outcomes. *J Refract Surg.* 2007;23(9 Suppl):S1029-S1036.
39. Fiore T, Carones F, Brancato R. Broad beam vs. flying spot excimer laser: refractive and videokeratographic outcomes of two different ablation profiles after photorefractive keratectomy. *J Refract Surg.* 2001;17:534-541.
40. Liang FQ, Ishikawa T, Kim J, Del Cerro M, Park SB, Aquavella JV. Surface quality of excimer laser corneal ablation with different frequencies. *Cornea.* 1993;12:500-506.
41. Fantes FE, Waring GO III. Effect of excimer laser radiant exposure on uniformity of ablated corneal surface. *Lasers Surg Med.* 1989;9:533-542.
42. Huang D, Arif M. Spot size and quality of scanning laser correction of higher-order wavefront aberrations. *J Cataract Refract Surg.* 2002;28:407-416.
43. Vinciguerra P, Azzolini M, Airaghi P, Radice P, De Molfetta V. Effect of decreasing surface and interface irregularities after photorefractive keratectomy and laser in situ keratomileusis on optical and functional outcomes. *J Refract Surg.* 1998;14:S199-S203.
44. Serrao S, Lombardo M. One-year results of photorefractive keratectomy with and without surface smoothing using the Technolas 217C laser. *J Refract Surg.* 2004;20:444-449.
45. Wilson SE. Molecular cell biology for the refractive corneal surgeon: programmed cell death and wound healing. *J Refract Surg.* 1997;13:171-175.
46. Nakamura Y, Sotozono C, Kinoshita S. The epidermal growth factor receptor (EGFR): role in corneal wound healing and homeostasis. *Exp Eye Res.* 2001;72:511-517.
47. Chandrasekher G, Ma X, Lallier TE, Bazan HEP. Delay of corneal epithelial wound healing and induction of keratocyte apoptosis by platelet-activating factor. *Invest Ophthalmol Vis Sci.* 2002;43:1422-1428.
48. Wilson S, Mohan RR, Hong JW, Lee JS, Choi R, Mohan RR. The wound healing response after laser in situ keratomileusis and photorefractive keratectomy. *Arch Ophthalmol.* 2001;119:889-896.
49. Gan L, Hamberg-Nystrom H, Fagerholm P, Van Setten G. Cellular proliferation and leukocyte infiltration in the rabbit cornea after photorefractive keratectomy. *Acta Ophthalmol Scand.* 2001;79:488.
50. Møller-Pedersen T, Cavanagh HD, Petroll WM, Jester JV. Stromal wound healing explains refractive instability and haze development after photorefractive keratectomy. *Ophthalmology.* 2000;107:1235-1245.
51. Fantes FE, Hanna KD, Waring III GO, Pouliquen Y, Thompson KP, Savoldelli M. Wound healing after excimer laser keratomileusis (photorefractive keratectomy) in monkeys. *Arch Ophthalmol.* 1990;108:665-675.
52. Jester JV , Møller-Pedersen T, Huang J. The cellular basis of corneal transparency: evidence for "corneal crystallins." *J Cell Sci.* 1999;112:613-622.
53. Amm M, Wetzel W, Winter M, Uthoff D, Duncker GIW. Histopathological comparison of photorefractive keratectomy and laser in situ keratomileusis in rabbits. *J Refract Surg.* 1996;12:758-766.
54. Nakamura K, Kurosaka D, Yoshiho M, Oshima T, Kurosaka H. Injured corneal epithelial cells promote myodifferentiation of corneal fibroblasts. *Invest Ophthalmol Vis Sci.* 2002;43:2603-2608.
55. Møller-Pedersen T, Li HF, Petroll WM, Cavanagh HD, Jester JV. Confocal microscopic characterization of wound repair after photorefractive keratectomy. *Invest Ophthalmol Vis Sci.* 1998;39:487-501.
56. Baldwin HC, Marshall J. Growth factors in corneal wound healing following refractive surgery: a review. *Acta Ophthalmol Scand.* 2002;80:238-247.

57. Moller-Pedersen T, Vogel M, Li HF, Petroll WM, Cavanagh HD, Jester JV. Quantification of stromal thinning, epithelial thickness, and corneal haze after photorefractive keratectomy using in vivo confocal microscopy. *Ophthalmology.* 1997;104:360-368.
58. Trokel SL, Srinivasan R, Braren B. Excimer laser surgery of the cornea. *Am J Ophthalmol.* 1983;96:710-715.
59. Lombardo M, De Santo MP, Lombardo G, Barberi R, Serrao S. Roughness of excimer laser ablated corneas with and without smoothing with atomic force microscopy. *J Refract Surg.* 2005;21:469-475.
60. Nogradi A, Hopp B, Revesz K, et al. Atomic force microscopic study of the human cornea following excimer laser keratectomy. *Exp Eye Res.* 2000;70:363-368.
61. Lydataki S, Lesniewska E, Tsilimbaris MK, Panagopoulou S, Le Grimellec G, Pallikaris IG. Excimer laser ablated cornea observed by atomic force microscopy. *Single Mol.* 2002;2-3:141-147.
62. Kerr-Muir MG, Trokel SL, Marshall J, Rothery S. Ultrastructural comparison of conventional surgical and argon fluoride excimer laser keratectomy. *Am J Ophthalmol.* 1987;103:448-453.
63. Maldonado-Codina C, Morgan PB, Efron N. Thermal consequences of photorefractive keratectomy. *Cornea.* 2001;20:509-515.
64. Betney S, Morgan PB, Doyle SJ, Efron N. Corneal temperature changes during photorefractive keratectomy. *Cornea.* 1997;16:158-161.
65. Thibos LN, Applegate RA, Schwiegereling JT, Webb R. VSIA Standards Taskforce Members. Standards for reporting the optical aberrations of eyes. *J Refract Surg.* 2002;18:S652-S660.
66. Thibos LN. Wavefront data reporting and terminology. *J Refract Surg.* 2001;17:S578-S583.
67. Applegate RA, Sarver EJ, Khemsara V. Are all aberrations equal? *J Refract Surg.* 2002;18:S556-S562.
68. Thibos LN, Hong X, Bradley A, Cheng X. Statistical variation of aberration structure and image quality in a normal population of healthy eyes. *J Opt Soc Am A Opt Image Sci Vis.* 2002;19:2329-2348.
69. Castejon-Mochon JF, Lopez-Gil N, Benito A, Artal P. Ocular wave-front aberration statistics in a normal young population. *Vision Res.* 2002;42:1611-1617.
70. Guirao A, Gonzalez C, Redondo M, Geraghty E, Norrby S, Artal P. Average optical performance of the human eye as a function of age in a normal population. *Invest Ophthalmol Vis Sci.* 1999;40:203-213.
71. Oshika T, Klyce SD, Applegate RA, Howland HC. Changes in corneal wavefront aberrations with aging. *Invest Ophthalmol Vis Sci.* 1999;40:1351-1355.
72. Lombardo M, Lombardo G. The wave aberration of human eyes and new descriptors of image optical quality of the eye. *J Cataract Refract Surg.* 2010;36:313-331.
73. Maurice DM, Monroe F. Cohesive strength of corneal lamellae. *Exp Eye Res.* 1990;50:59-63.
74. Smolek MK, McCarey BE. Interlamellar adhesive strength in human eye bank corneas. *Invest Ophthalmol Vis Sci.* 1990;31:1087-1095.
75. Smolek MK. Interlamellar cohesive strength in the vertical meridian of human eye bank corneas. *Invest Ophthalmol Vis Sci.* 1993;34:2962-2969.
76. Hedbys BO, Dohlman CH. A new method for the determination of the swelling pressure of the corneal stroma in vitro. *Exp Eye Res.* 1963;2:122-129.
77. Katsube N. The constitutive theory of fluid-filled porous materials. *J Applied Mech.* 1985;52:185-189.
78. Katsube N, Wang R, Okuma E, Roberts C. Biomechanical response of the cornea to phototherapeutic keratectomy when treated as a fluid-filled porous material. *J Refract Surg.* 2002;18:S593-S597.
79. Roberts C. The cornea is not a piece of plastic. *J Refract Surg.* 2000;16:407-413.
80. Dupps WJ, Roberts C, Schoessler JP. Peripheral lamellar relaxation: a mechanism of induced corneal flattening in PTK and PRK? *Invest Ophthalmol Vis Sci.* 1995;36:S708.
81. Roorda A, Metha AB, Lennie P, Williams DR. Packing arrangement of the three cone classes in primate retina. *Vision Res.* 2001;41:1291-1306.
82. Roorda A. Adaptive optics ophthalmoscopy. *J Refract Surg.* 2000;16:S602-S607.
83. Le Gargasson JF, Glanc M, Lena P. Retinal imaging with adaptive optics. *Biophysics.* 2001:1131-1138.
84. Fernandez EJ, Manzanera S, Piers P, Artal P. Adaptive optics visual simulator. *J Refract Surg.* 2002;18:S634-S638.
85. Fiore T, Carones F, Brancato R. Broad beam vs. flying spot excimer laser: refractive and videokeratographic outcomes of two different ablation profiles after photorefractive keratectomy. *J Refract Surg.* 2001;17:534-540.
86. Fagerholm P. Phototherapeutic keratectomy: 12 years of experience. *Acta Ophthalmol Scand.* 2003;81:19-32.
87. Kornmehl EW, Steinert RF, Puliafito CA. A comparative study of masking fluids for excimer laser phototherapeutic keratectomy. *Arch Ophthalmol.* 1991;109:860-863.
88. Serrao S, Lombardo M, Mondini F. Photorefractive keratectomy with and without smoothing: a bilateral study. *J Refract Surg.* 2003;19:58-64.
89. Steele JG, Johnson G, McLean KM, Beumer GJ, Griesser HJ. Effect of porosity and surface hydrophilicity on migration of epithelial tissue over synthetic polymer. *J Biomed Mater Res.* 2000;50:475-482.
90. Horgan SE, McLaughlin-Borlace L, Stevens JD, Munro PMG. Phototherapeutic smoothing as an adjunct to photorefractive keratectomy in porcine cornea. *J Refract Surg.* 1999;15:331-333.
91. Serrao S, Lombardo G, Lombardo M, Palombi M, Roberts C. Corneal topography six years after photorefractive keratectomy for myopia and myopic astigmatism. *J Refract Surg.* 2009;25:451-458.
92. Lombardo M, Lombardo G, Manzulli M, Serrao S. Response of the cornea for up to four-years after photorefractive keratectomy. *J Refract Surg.* 2006;22:178-186.
93. Wigledowska-Promienska D, Zawojska I. Changes in higher order aberrations after wavefront-guided PRK for correction of low to moderate myopia and myopic astigmatism: two-year follow-up. *Eur J Ophthalmol.* 2007;17:507-514.
94. Shojaei A, Mohammad-Rabei H, Eslani M, Elahi B, Noorizadeh F. Long-term evaluation of complications and results of photorefractive keratectomy in myopia: an 8-year follow-up. *Cornea.* 2009;28:304-310.
95. Koch DD, Kohnen T, Obstbaum SA, Rosen ES. Format for reporting refractive surgical data. *J Cataract Refract Surg.* 1998;24:285-287.

96. Maloney RK, Bogan SJ, Waring GO III. Determination of corneal image-forming properties from corneal topography. *Am J Ophthalmol.* 1993;115:31-41.
97. Einighammer J, Oltrup T, Bende T, Jean B. Real ray tracing simulation versus clinical outcomes of corneal excimer laser surface ablations. *J Refract Surg.* 2010;e-published.
98. Munnerlyn CR, Koons SJ, Marshall J. Photorefractive keratectomy: a technique for laser refractive surgery. *J Cataract Refract Surg.* 1988;14:46-52.
99. Mrochen M, Kaemmerer M, Mierdel P, Seiler T. Increased higher-order optical aberrations after laser refractive surgery. A problem of subclinical decentration. *J Cataract Refract Surg.* 2001;27:362-369.
100. Oliver KM, O'Brart DPS, Stephenson CG, et al. Anterior corneal optical aberrations induced by photorefractive keratectomy for hyperopia. *J Refract Surg.* 2001;17: 406-413.
101. Vinciguerra P, Sborgia M, Epstein D, Azzolini M, MacRae S. Photorefractive keratectomy to correct myopic or hyperopic astigmatism with a cross-cylinder ablation. *J Refract Surg.* 1999;15:S183-S185.
102. Chayet AS, Magallanes R, Montes M, Chavez S, Robledo N. Laser in situ keratomileusis for simple myopic, mixed and simple hyperopic astigmatism. *J Refract Surg.* 1998;14: S175-S176.
103. Schwiegerling J, Snyder R. Corneal ablation patterns to correct for spherical aberration in photorefractive keratectomy. *J Cataract Refract Surg.* 2000;26:214-221.
104. Mejia-Barbosa Y, Malacara-Hernandez D. A review of methods for measuring corneal topography. *Opt Vis Sci.* 2001;78:240-253.
105. Campin JA, Pettit GH, Gray GP. Required laser beam resolution and PRK system configuration for custom high fidelity corneal shaping. *Invest Ophthalmol Vis Sci.* 1999;38:S538.
106. Mrochen M, Eldine MS, Kaemmer M, Seile T, Hütz W. Improvement in photorefractive corneal laser surgery results using an active eye-tracking system. *J Cataract Refract Surg.* 2001;27:1000-1006.
107. Koch DD, Maloney R, Hardten DR, Dell S, Sweeney AD, Wang L. Wavefront-guided photorefractive keratectomy in eyes with prior radial keratotomy: a multicenter study. *Ophthalmology.* 2009;116:1688-1696.
108. Mastropasqua L, Toto L, Zuppardi E, et al. Zyoptix wavefront-guided versus standard photorefractive keratectomy (PRK) in low and moderate myopia: randomized controlled 6-month study. *Eur J Ophthalmol.* 2006;16: 219-228.
109. Karimian F, Feizi S, Jafarinasab MR. Conventional versus custom ablation in photorefractive keratectomy: randomized clinical trial. *J Cataract Refract Surg.* 2010;36: 637-643.
110. Ghoreishi SM, Naderibeni A, Peyman A, Rismanchian A, Eslami F. Aspheric profile versus wavefront-guided ablation photorefractive keratectomy for the correction of myopia using the Allegretto Eye Q. *Eur J Ophthalmol.* 2009;19:544-553.
111. Falavarjani KG, Hashemi M, Modarres M, Sanjari MS, Darvish N, Gordiz A. Topography-guided vs wavefront-optimized surface ablation for myopia using the WaveLight platform: a contralateral eye study. *J Refract Surg.* 2010;19:1-5.
112. Vinciguerra P, Albè E, Camesasca FI, Trazza S, Epstein D. Wavefront- versus topography-guided customized ablations with the NIDEK EC-5000 CX II in surface ablation treatment: refractive and aberrometric outcomes. *J Refract Surg.* 2007;23(9 Suppl):S1029-S1036.
113. Kermani O, Schmiedt K, Oberheide U, Gerten G. Topographic- and wavefront-guided customized ablations with the NIDEK-EC5000CXII in LASIK for myopia. *J Refract Surg.* 2006;22:754-763.
114. Weber BA, Gan L, Fagerholm PP. Short-term impact of corticosteroids on hyaluronan and epithelial hyperplasia in the rabbit cornea after photorefractive keratectomy. *Cornea.* 2001;20:321-324.
115. Price FW Jr, Willes L, Price M, Lyng A, Ries J. A prospective, randomized comparison of the use versus non-use of topical corticosteroids after laser in situ keratomileusis. *Ophthalmology.* 2001;108:1236-1244.
116. Lipshitz I. Thirty-four challenges to meet before excimer laser technology can achieve super vision. *J Refract Surg.* 2002;18:740-743.
117. Yap EY, Kowal L. Diplopia as a complication of laser in situ keratomileusis surgery. *Clin Experiment Ophthalmol.* 2001;29:268-271.

Part II

Photorefractive Keratectomy Enhancement Following Previous Radial Keratotomy and LASIK

Mounir A. Khalifa, MD, PhD and Waleed A. Allam, MD, PhD

Photorefractive keratectomy (PRK) involves ablation of the corneal stroma on its surface. The Food and Drug Administration approved PRK for myopia in 1995[1] and later for hyperopia and astigmatism.

During the past 2 decades, many studies have shown the safety and efficacy of PRK as a primary procedure for correction of refractive errors in virgin eyes,[2] as well as an enhancement procedure for correction of residual errors after previous refractive and/or corneal surgeries.[3] This chapter highlights the practical aspects of the use of PRK for enhancement of residual errors after radial keratotomy (RK) and laser in situ keratomileusis (LASIK).

Indications for enhancements include primary over- and/or under-correction, induced or residual astigmatism, and regression over time. RK patients with very small central zones (clear of incisions) or with incisions extending inside the central cornea and optical axis (Figures 4-1 and 4-2) may have reduced optical quality with night vision complaints due to higher-order aberrations (HOAs). These may be able to be addressed by enhancements using wavefront-guided ablation. Similarly, LASIK patients with de-centered ablations, steep central islands, and intraoperative flap complications such as small flaps, buttonholes, and torn flaps may benefit from enhancements with PRK. It's worth noting that the proper timing for PRK enhancement depends on the specific indication as well as the refractive stability. Generally speaking, refractive stability can be obtained somewhere around 3 months after the primary procedure, depending on the actual primary surgery.

Treatment Plan

PRK enhancement of previous RK and LASIK patients is simple and straightforward in many cases. However, there are specific cases that present with challenges. In some patients with irregular astigmatism and large amounts of HOAs, obtaining consistent manifest refractions and wavefront maps may not be possible. Consequently, the treatment plan may have to be based on what is available:

1. *Plan 1:* Regular corneas on topography with consistent manifest refraction and reliable wavefront maps. These patients are the typical candidates for wavefront-guided treatments.
2. *Plan 2:* Regular corneas on topography with consistent manifest refraction but without a reliable wavefront map. For these patients, we recommend conventional treatments, such as optimized ablation profiles to correct the residual error with less induction of additional spherical aberrations.

Buratto L, Slade S, Serrao S, Lombardo M. ***PRK: The Past, Present, and Future of Surface Ablation.*** *(pp. 65-70).*

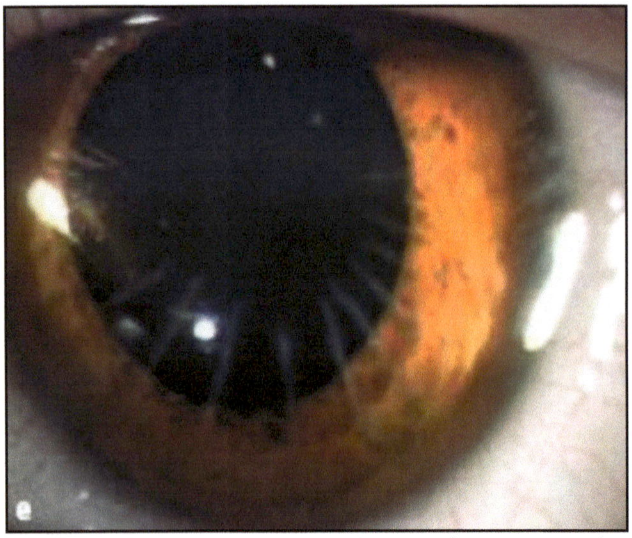

Figure 4-1. Asymmetric RK incisions resulting in irregular astigmatism.

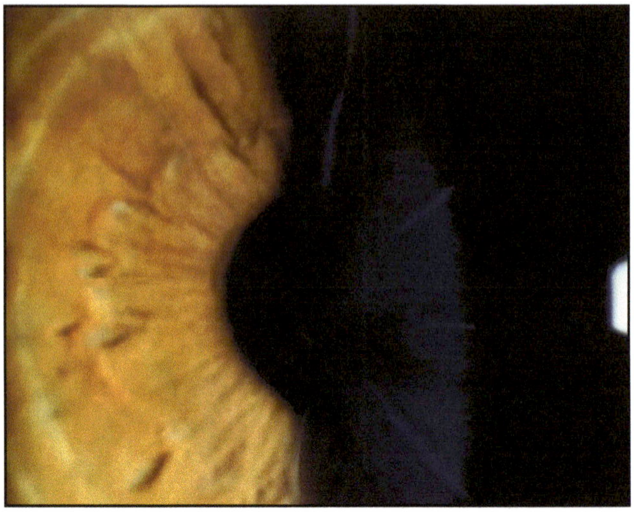

Figure 4-2. Small optical zone with RK incisions inside the central corneal area.

3. *Plan 3:* A consistent manifest refraction, but irregular cornea on topography and no available reliable wavefront map. One-step topography-guided ablation is the recommended approach for such cases (Figures 4-3A and B).
4. *Plan 4:* Irregular corneas on topography and neither consistent manifest refraction nor reliable wavefront mapping. Two-step topography-guided ablation works best with such cases. In the first step, we use the laser to just smooth out the cornea, aiming at reducing the irregularities and making refraction possible. While the second step aims at refractive correction.

In our opinion, the best enhancements are obtained with wavefront-guided ablation from a reliable wavefront map.

Mitomycin C

Mitomycin C (MMC) is a systemic alkylating chemotherapeutic agent with both cytotoxic and anti-proliferative effects that reduce myofibroblast repopulation after laser surface ablation. Mitomycin may reduce subepithelial haze formation. Although this use has not yet been approved by the FDA, MMC has been used both prophylactically to avoid subepithelial haze associated with primary surface ablation[4] and therapeutically to treat cases with already pre-existing haze.[5]

In our hands, we routinely apply MMC at a concentration of 0.2 mg/mL (0.02 mg%) in all cases of PRK enhancements after RK or LASIK, regardless of the amount of the correction. A 6-mm sponge soaked with MMC is applied to the ablated zone of the cornea for 30 seconds to 2 minutes (Figure 4-4), after which the cornea is thoroughly irrigated using balanced salt solution.

PRK After Previous LASIK

PRK vs LASIK

Enhancements of previous LASIK patients may be performed with either PRK or LASIK (flap lift or new cut),[6] depending on the individual indication as well as the intended correction. A flap lift technique is our preferred approach to enhance previous uneventful LASIK (eg, cases with simple under- and/or over-corrections). We prefer surface ablation on top of previous LASIK flaps if there are concerns about the residual stromal bed thickness (RBT). Cases with intraoperative LASIK flap complications, such as buttonholes and small or incomplete flaps, may be treated by either PRK or cutting new larger and thicker flaps after an appropriate time interval.

Technique

Two main concerns related to performing surface ablation on top of previous LASIK flaps are the appropriate method of corneal epithelial removal

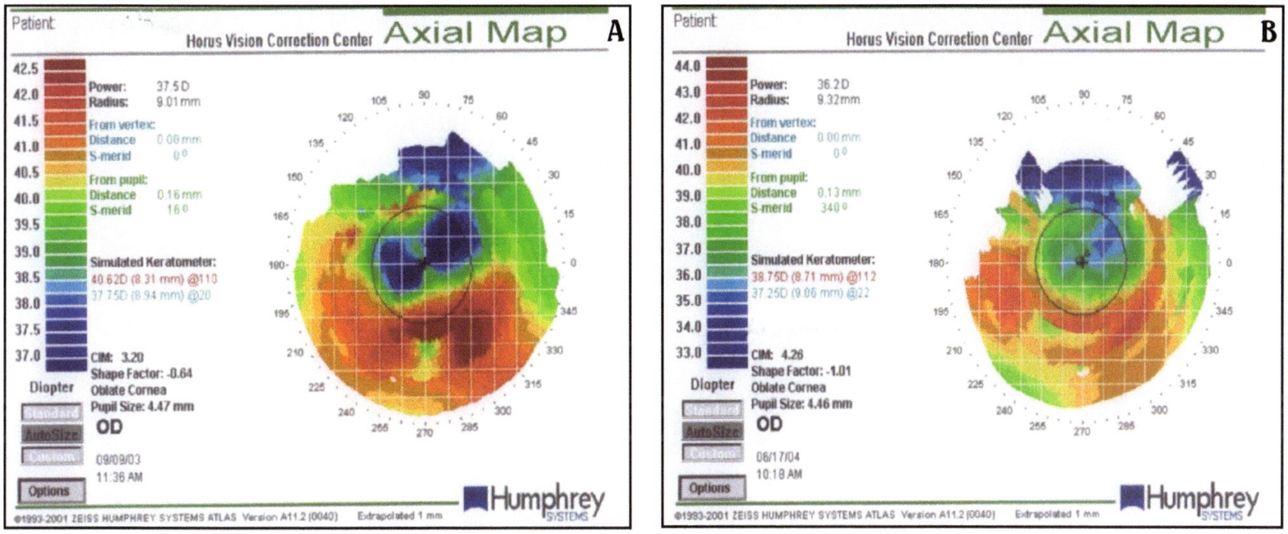

Figure 4-3. RK patient before (A) and 9 months after (B) topography-guided PRK enhancement with MMC.

and prophylaxis against possible postoperative haze formation.

In previously unoperated eyes, the epithelium may be removed by several methods, including mechanical (scraping or rotating brush) and laser scrape (trans-epithelial PRK) techniques. Removing the epithelium on a previous LASIK flap should be either mechanically assisted by alcohol or by laser scrape.[7] Purely mechanical means of epithelial removal should be avoided, as they might threaten the smoothness and adherence of the flap.

Alcohol-assisted epithelial removal is best accomplished by applying a 9-mm optical zone marker to the surface of the cornea centered on the visual axis, with gentle pressure, to score the epithelium at the edge of the marker. A few drops of ethyl alcohol 20% solution are dropped onto the surface of the cornea, keeping the marker in place as a well, immersing the whole area inside the well. The alcohol is thus held in place 25 to 30 seconds, then removed with microsurgical spears while the marker is in place to avoid leakage of the solution onto the limbal and conjunctival epithelium. The remaining alcohol should be thoroughly irrigated with balanced salt solution. At that time, the epithelium is loose enough to be removed by gentle strokes using a 15 blade. The strokes should start at the hinge location and gently go away from the hinge so as to not jeopardize flap adherence.

Trans-epithelial PRK[7] is another option available in laser platforms such as the Visx STAR S4 (Visx, Santa Clara, CA). The machine is set to an ablation depth of 50 μm, which is enough to ablate the epithelium in most cases. A characteristic fluorescence, in dim room light, may be observed during excimer laser ablation to the epithelium. Cessation of this fluorescence is the practical endpoint, indicating complete removal of the epithelium.

PRK After Previous RK

Many post-RK patients report diurnal vision fluctuations. The Prospective Evaluation of Radial Keratotomy (PERK) Study showed that such fluctuations last for at least 11 years after the primary procedure. According to the study, 51% of eyes showed an increase in minus power of manifest refraction of 0.5 to 1.62 D and a central corneal steepening of 0.5 to 1.94 D during the day.[8] This indicates that corneal stability might not be attained during the first 11 years after RK, a fact that must be considered when evaluating RK patients for enhancements. The exact cause of this phenomenon is still unknown; however, it may be related to structural integrity changes and incomplete healing of the corneal RK incisions.

PRK/RK Technique Points

Careful mechanical removal of the epithelium should be carried out with special attention to completely remove the raised epithelial plugs at the incision sites. Alcohol may facilitate this step. After performing the ablation, MMC is applied for 30 seconds to 2 minutes to reduce the incidence of haze as mentioned before.

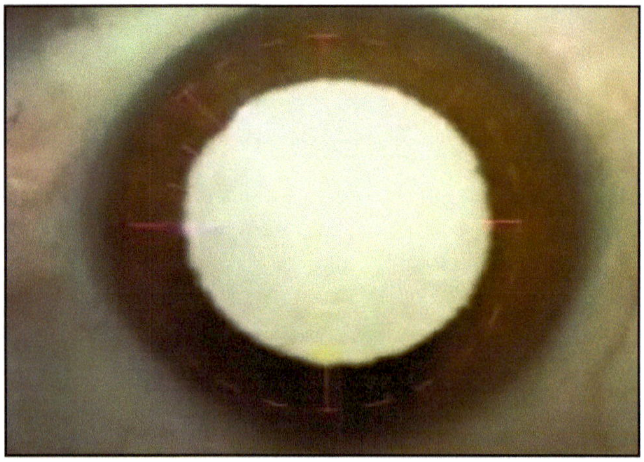

Figure 4-4. Application of MMC after PRK ablation.

PRK vs LASIK

As with many enhancement procedures, the selection of a particular technique is very case-dependent. In 2010, we studied the results of PRK with MMC vs LASIK (in 18 and 21 eyes, respectively) for enhancements after RK using wavefront-guided ablation of the Visx STAR S4. Both techniques were effective in correcting residual errors after RK; however, the LASIK group showed a higher safety index (ratio of the postoperative best-corrected visual acuity [BCVA] to the preoperative BCVA) due to the development of visually significant haze in 12% of PRK eyes. A significant improvement in total HOAs, coma, and spherical aberrations was observed in both groups. Trefoil aberrations were reduced more in the PRK eyes (Figure 4-5). Point spread function showed significant improvement after wavefront-guided ablation in both PRK and LASIK cases (Figure 4-6).[9]

The creation of the flap is a major concern when performing LASIK after RK. Cutting through the previous RK incisions relaxes the tension at the scar lines with possible changes in the refraction due to the induced corneal shape changes. We thus recommend LASIK after RK to be done in two stages: flap creation, then laser ablation 3 months later. Also, RK scars may be disrupted during the flap creation, leading to poor flap quality and an increased risk for subsequent epithelial ingrowth. Finally, as in any decision whether to do LASIK or PRK, corneal thickness also should be considered during the decision-making.

References

1. Hersh PS, Stulting RD, Steinert RF, et al. Results of phase III excimer laser photorefractive keratectomy for myopia. The Summit PRK study group. *Ophthalmology.* 1997;104:1535-1553.
2. Bababeygy SR, Manche EE. Wavefront-guided photorefractive keratectomy with the VISX platform for myopia. *J Refract Surg.* 2010;28:1-8.
3. Alio JL, Pinero DP, Plaza Puche AB. Corneal wavefront-guided photorefractive keratectomy in patients with irregular corneas after corneal refractive surgery. *J Cataract Refract Surg.* 2008;34:1727-1735.
4. Carones F, Vigo L, Scandola E, et al. Evaluation of the prophylactic use of mitomycin-C to inhibit haze formation after photorefractive keratectomy. *J Cataract Refract Surg.* 2002;28:2088-2095.
5. Majmudar PA, Forstot SL, Dennis RF, et al. Topical mitomycin-C for subepithelial fibrosis after refractive corneal surgery. *Ophthalmology.* 2000;107:89-94.
6. Davis EA, Hardten DR, Lindstrom M, et al. LASIK enhancements: A comparison of lifting to recutting the flap. *Ophthalmology.* 2002;109:2308-2313.
7. Muller LT, Candal EM, Epstein RJ, et al. Transepithelial phototherapeutic keratectomy/photorefractive keratectomy with adjunctive mitomycin-C for complicated LASIK flaps. *J Cataract Refract Surg.* 2005;31:291-296.
8. McDonell PJ, Nizam A, Lynn MJ, et al. Morning to evening change in refraction, corneal curvature, and visual acuity 11 years after radial keratotomy in the Prospective Evaluation of Radial Keratotomy study. *Ophthalmology.* 1996;103:233-239.
9. Khalifa MA. Wavefront-guided LASIK versus PRK after radial keratotomy. Presented at the American Society of Cataract and Refractive Surgery meeting, San Diego, March 2011.

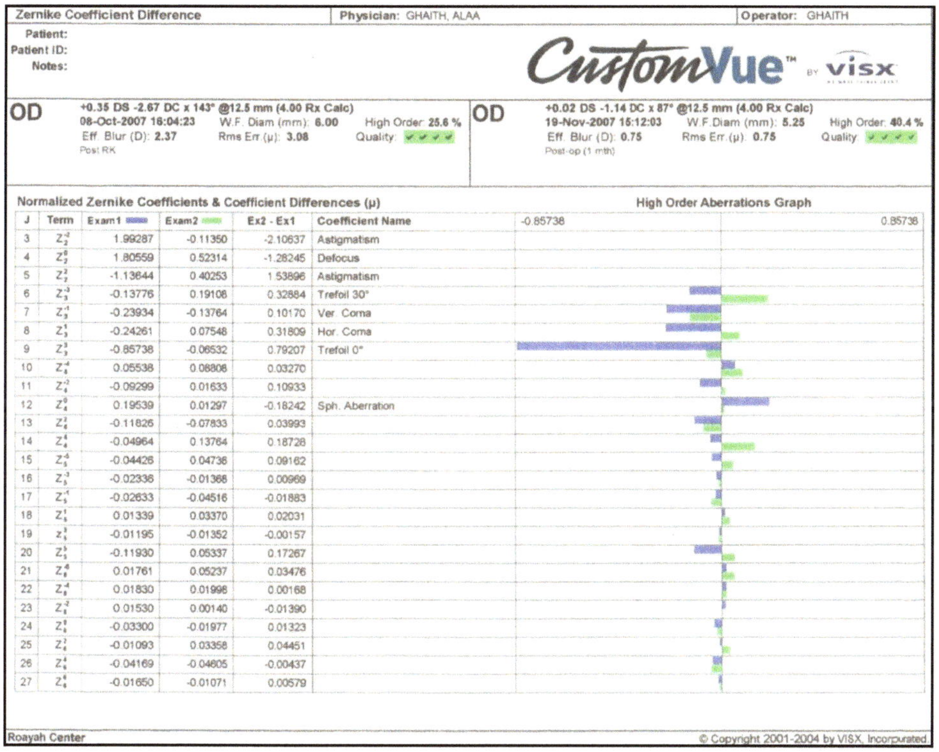

Figure 4-5. Zernike coefficient difference before and 6 weeks after wavefront-guided PRK enhancement of previous RK.

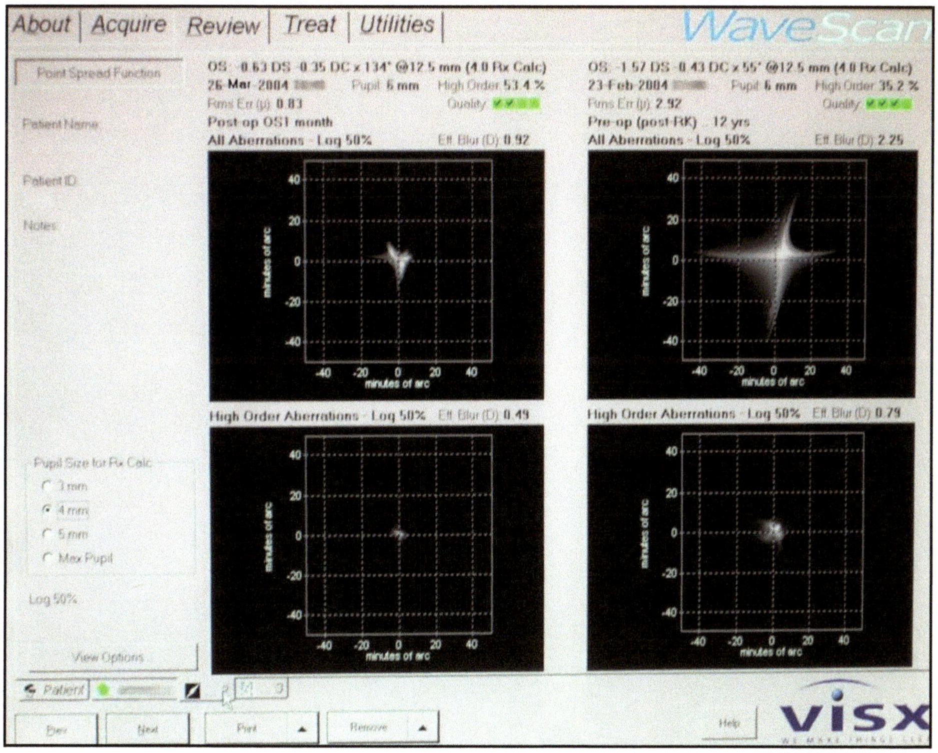

Figure 4-6. PSF before and 4 weeks after wavefront-guided PRK enhancement of previous RK.

Chapter 5

Smoothing in Refractive Surgery

Paolo Vinciguerra, MD; Elena Albé, MD; and R. Vinciguerra, MD

The quality of the ablation surface is critical....

It is well-known that extremely important factors for successful photoablation include the creation of a regular corneal profile with a low gradient and without sharp and abrupt changes in curvature. These irregular curvature changes may induce an excessive reparative response of the epithelium with increased deposition of collagen, reduce the desired refractive effect, and induce corneal aberrations.

Refractive surgery may often lead to inconsistent results due to saccadic eye motion and loss of fixation during the procedure, even in the presence of an advanced eye-tracking system. Unreliable results may also be due to the individual patient's corneal reparative response and corneal healing, which can seldom be modulated by postoperative pharmacological treatment.

In addition, different types of excimer lasers have a different influence on the final result according to their beam shape or ablation geometry. Each ablation pattern (broad beam, flying spot, etc) induces a moderate surface irregularity, resulting from the overlap of each spot. No currently available laser beam impacts the cornea with a uniform pattern nor is capable of creating a perfect surface without leaving small, unexposed areas, resulting in an irregular surface. This irregularity increases with the amount of diopters that are treated during the excimer laser procedure (Figures 5-1 and 5-2).

A slit-lamp examination highlights only the major irregularities.[1-2] Digitalized retro-illumination with a Scheimpflug camera device may provide us with a better understanding of the corneal smoothness at the surface and at the stromal interface level 1. Each tiny irregularity induces light diffraction caused by light passing through media with different refraction indices thus deviated from its original linear direction. A corneal surface irregularity scale may be established and evaluated intraoperatively immediately after photoablation (Figure 5-3).

- Grade I: No irregularities (Figure 5-4).
- Grade II: Moderate irregularities (Figure 5-5).
- Grade III: Severe irregularities (Figure 5-6).

Irregularities larger than 50 μm induce collagen deposition with an unpredictable refractive outcome. A more regular surface typically stimulates the reparative process less and may alter the refractive result to a lesser degree, diminishing regression and haze.[3-5] As Netto and colleagues demonstrated in their original paper, there is a relationship between the level of corneal haze formation after PRK and the level of stromal surface irregularity.[6] More collagen deposition means more reduction in the induced refractive effect, often in an unpredictable pattern (Figure 5-7).

Buratto L, Slade S, Serrao S, Lombardo M. ***PRK: The Past, Present, and Future of Surface Ablation.*** ***(pp. 71-76).***

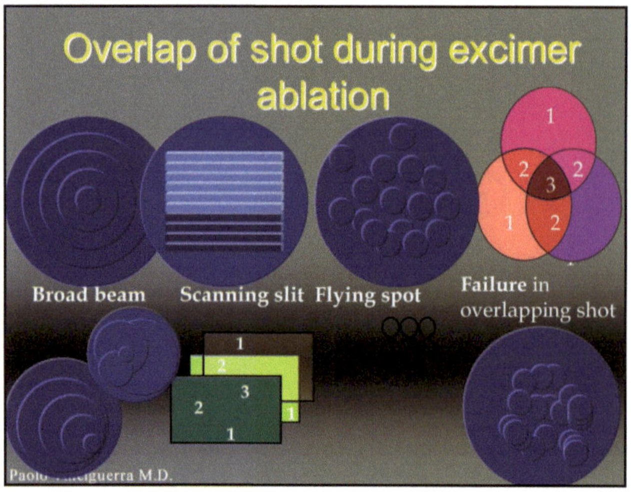

Figure 5-1. Examples of shot overlapping during excimer ablation.

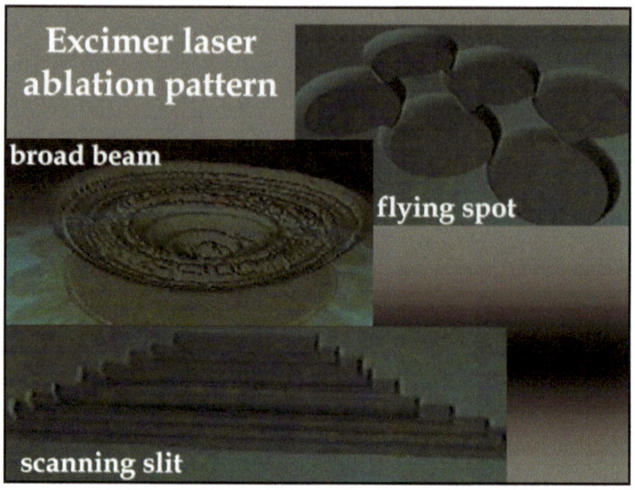

Figure 5-2. Different excimer laser ablation pattern.

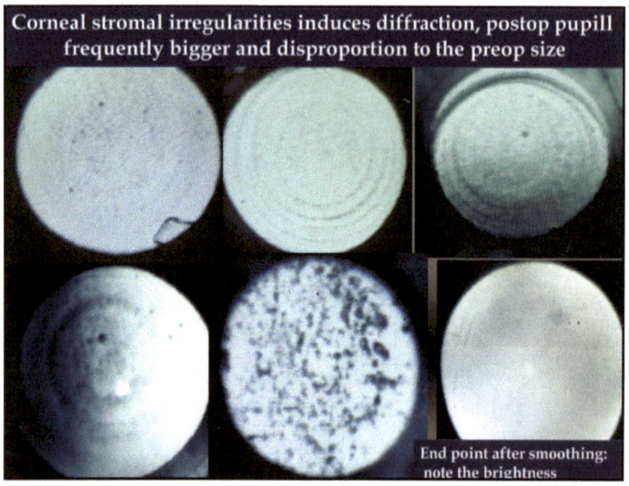

Figure 5-3. Corneal stromal irregularities due to shot overlapping during excimer ablation.

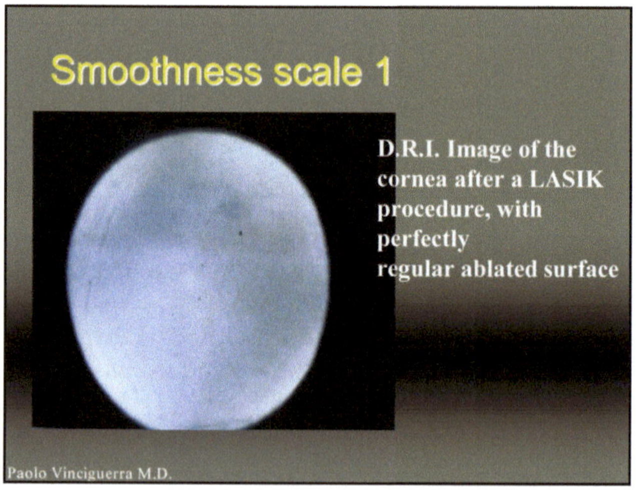

Figure 5-4. Transilluminated cornea resembling smoothness scale 1.

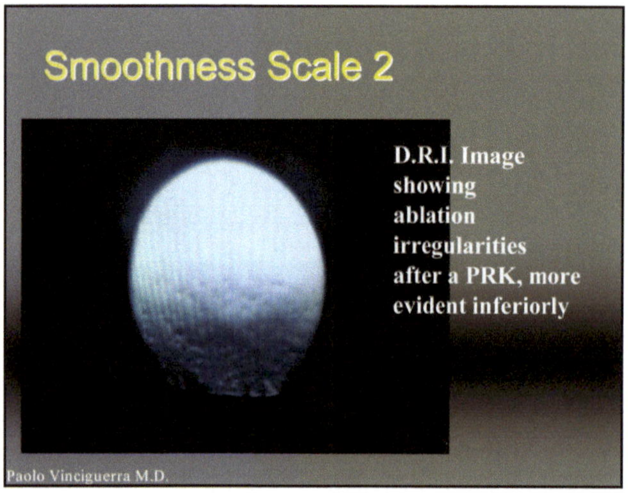

Figure 5-5. Transilluminated cornea resembling smoothness scale 2.

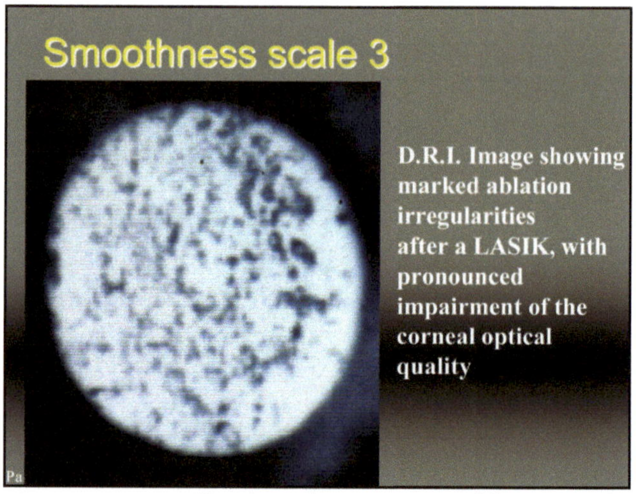

Figure 5-6. Transilluminated cornea resembling smoothness scale 3.

References

1. Vinciguerra P, Azzolini M, Radice P, Sborgia M, Molfetta V. A method for examining surface and interface irregularities after photorefractive keratectomy and laser in situ keratomileusis: predictor of optical and functional outcomes. *J Refract Surg.* 1998;14:S204-S206.
2. Vinciguerra, Azzolini M, Airaghi P, Radice P, de Molfetta V. Effect of decreasing surface and interface irregularities after photorefractive keratectomy and laser in situ keratomileusis on optical and functional outcomes. *J Refract Surg.* 1998;14:S199-S203.
3. Lombardo M, De Santo MP, Lombardo G, Barberi R, Serrao S. Roughness of excimer laser ablated corneas with and without smoothing measured with atomic force microscopy. *J Refract Surg.* 2005;21:469-475.
4. Serrao S, Lombardo M, Mondini F. Photorefractive keratectomy with and without smoothing: a bilateral study. *J Refract Surg.* 2003;19:58-64.
5. Serrao S, Lombardo M. Corneal epithelial healing after photorefractive keratectomy: analytical study. *J Cataract Refract Surg.* 2005;31:930-937.
6. Netto MV, Mohan RR, Sinha S, Sharma A, Dupps W, Wilson SE. Stromal haze, myofibroblasts, and surface irregularity after PRK. *Exp Eye Res.* 2006:82:788-797.
7. Kornhehl EW, Steinert RF, Puliafito CA. A comparative study of masking fluids for excimer laser phototherapeutic keratectomy. *Arch Ophthalmol.* 1991;109:860-863.
8. Vinciguerra P, Cro M, Giuffrida S, Airaghi P, de Molfetta V. A new strategy in excimer laser PTK: use of hyaluronic acid solution as masking fluid. *Inv Ophthalmol Vis Sci.* Annual Meeting, Sarasota, FL, May 1-6, 1994.
9. Fasano AP, Moreira M, McDonnell PJ, Sanbawy A. Excimer laser smoothing of a reproducible model of anterior corneal surface irregularity. *Ophthalmology.* 1991;98:1782-1785.
10. Vinciguerra P, Munoz MI, Camesasca FI, Grizzi F, Roberts C. Long-term follow-up of ultrathin corneas after surface retreatment with phototherapeutic keratectomy. *J Cataract Refract Surg.* 2005;31:82-87.

Chapter 6

How to Perform Custom Ablation

Paolo Vinciguerra, MD; Elena Albé, MD; and R. Vinciguerra, MD

Custom ablations, either based on surface topography, total aberrometry, or ray tracing, have raised interest among refractive surgeons for the potential to personalize each patient's correction. Such customized ablations aim at optimizing the optical system and unmasking and correcting the actual sphero-cylindrical error through the recognition and ablation of higher-order aberrations.

Custom Ablation Transition Zone software performed by the Final Fit Program of the NIDEK EC5000 excimer laser (Gamagori, Japan) optimizes the treatment of the ocular aberrations detected in the 4.5-mm central zone, particularly spherical aberrations. The curvature of the remaining cornea is then gradually modified in order to achieve a constant curvature gradient up to the external 10 mm margin of the ablation. This attempts to produce the highest possible reduction of ocular aberrations. The ablation plan includes an aspherical component for treatment of spherical defects (radial symmetrical aberrations), a toric component for treatment of astigmatism (linearly symmetric aberrations), and a flying spot component for the treatment of higher-order aberrations (irregular components).

The Final Fit program may offer a major advantage compared to other excimer laser ablation software. It doesn't show the actual portion of tissue that the laser plans to remove to correct the refractive error, but simulates the real shape after the planned tissue removal. This simulation gives the surgeon the opportunity to check the corneal regularity and shape with different kinds of maps (instantaneous, axial, refractive, etc) during each step of the ablation plan, with continuous feedback from the actual amount of tissue removed to obtain a more precise result of the final shape of the cornea.

Ablation Steps

1. Because the typical astigmatism has a higher-order aberration (HOA) component, the HOAs must be first corrected before the true astigmatism can be identified. The portion of the ablation for the higher-order aberration component is thus applied first. Higher-order corneal surface aberrations, which are naturally irregular and asymmetric, influence the cylinder power and axis measured preoperatively. The correction of higher-order aberrations may reveal the true cylinder power and axis, eliminating the coma and trefoil-related portion of astigmatism, as shown in Figure 6-1.
2. In this example, the new topographical axis and power of the astigmatism have been estimated and properly corrected. What looks like an irregular astigmatism may actually be a

Buratto L, Slade S, Serrao S, Lombardo M. ***PRK: The Past, Present, and Future of Surface Ablation.*** *(pp. 77-80).*

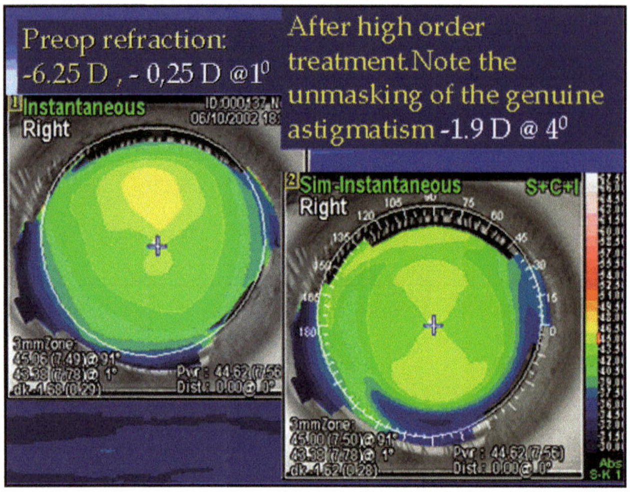

Figure 6-1. Astigmatism unmasked by high-order aberration treatment.

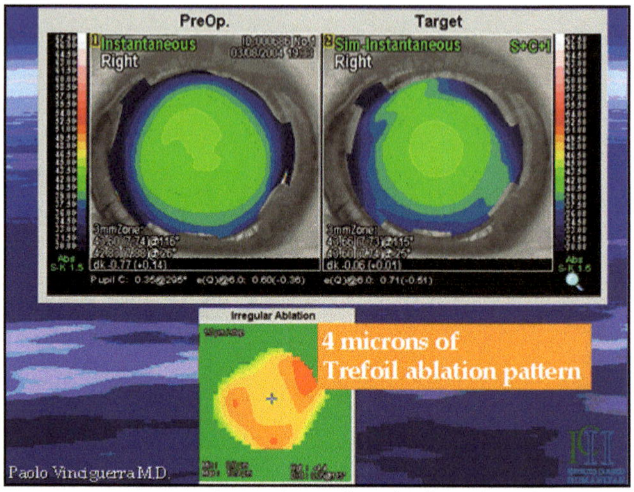

Figure 6-2. No astigmatism after high-order aberration treatment.

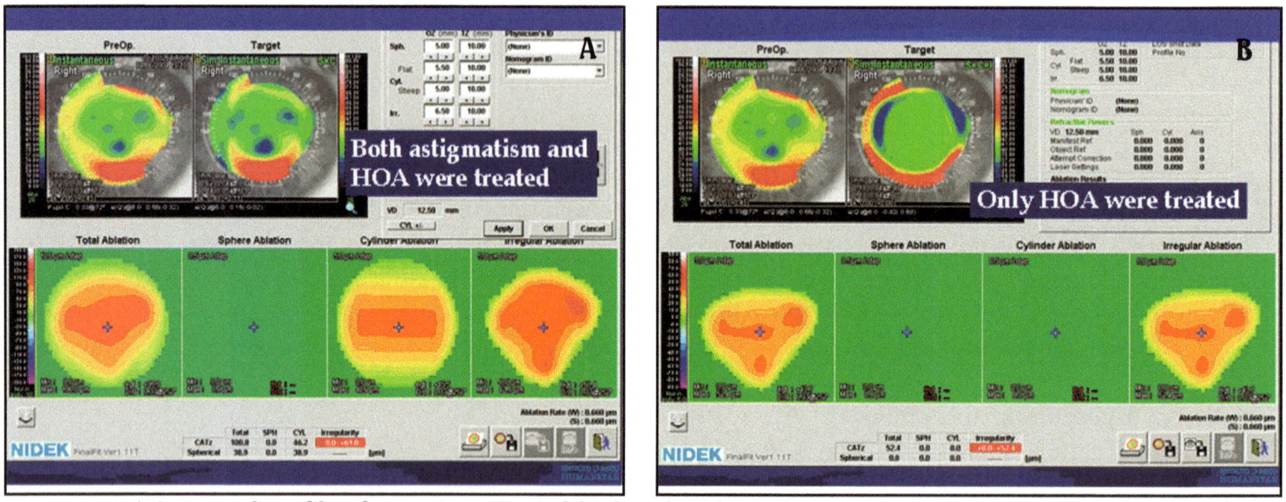

Figure 6-3. (A) Corneal profile after astigmatic and high-order aberration treatment. (B) Corneal profile after high-order aberration treatment.

combination of HOAs. After those aberrations are treated, it may turn out that there is actually no astigmatism (Figure 6-2). An example of an irregular cornea is shown in Figure 6-3A. Both cylinder and irregular components were treated with a removal of more than 60 μm of tissue. In Figure 6-3B, the same cornea is treated only by HOA component removal. As the target-simulated instantaneous topography shows, the final cornea becomes more regular with additional corneal tissue sparing.

Figure 6-4 shows another example in which treating the higher-order errors changes the axis of the unmasked astigmatism.

3. The final resulting spherical component to be treated is calculated.

If we were to ignore the facts explained above, poorly tolerated visual conditions could result for the patient, including the following:

- Pseudo-decentration (Figure 6-5).
- Residual astigmatism (Figure 6-6).
- Induction of new higher-order errors as errors in determining axis are usually coupled to power errors (Figure 6-7).
- Residual refractive error (see Figure 6-6).
- Poor vision.

This method has several advantages:

- To reduce the amount of tissue ablated, shorten ablation times, and redistribute the amount of removed tissue over the total corneal surface to preserve the biomechanical corneal strength.

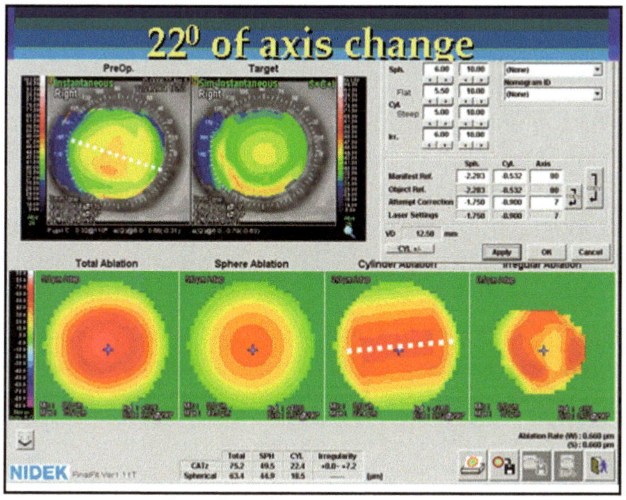

Figure 6-4. High-order aberration treatment changes the axis of remaining astigmatism.

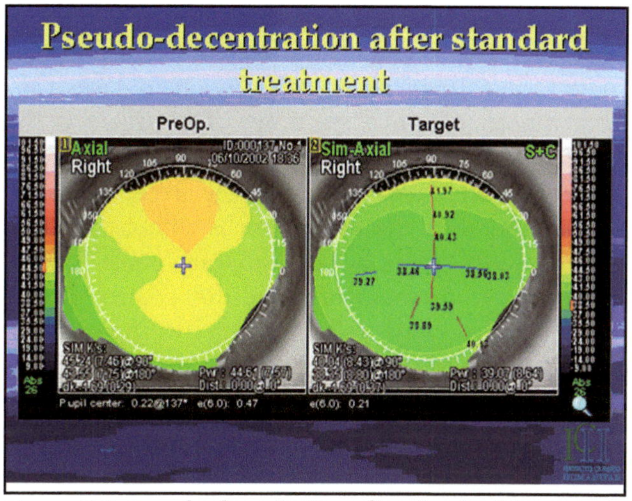

Figure 6-5. Pseudo-decentration after standard treatment.

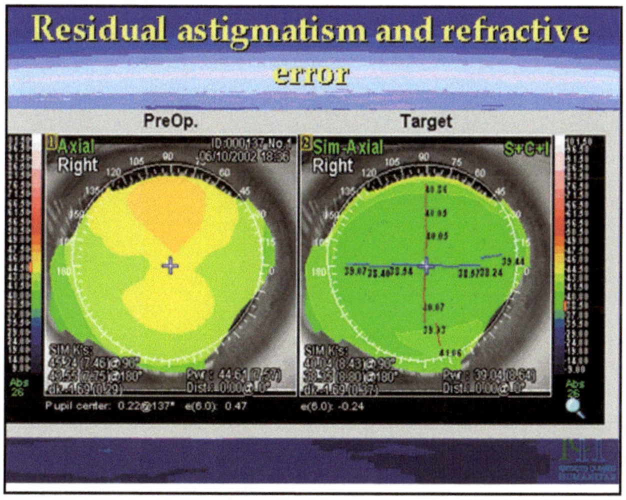

Figure 6-6. Residual astigmatism and refractive error after standard treatment.

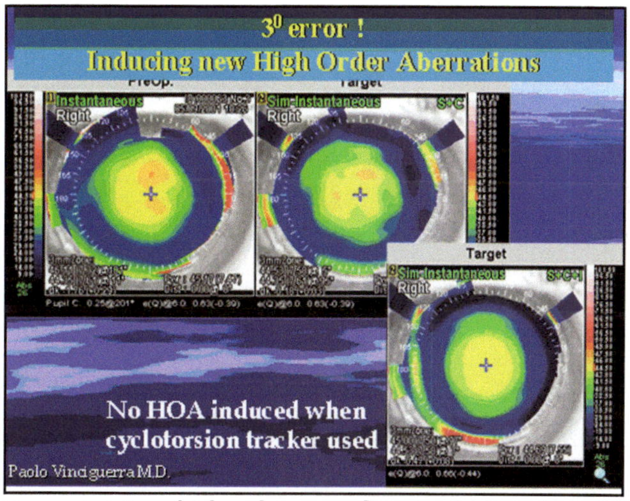

Figure 6-7. New high-order error after standard treatment.

- A more consistent final corneal curvature gradient with a reduction of the curvature gradient from the center to the periphery, especially in the extreme periphery, beyond 9 mm, where the cornea is thicker and flatter. This induces a further reduction of the spherical aberration to improve the quality of vision particularly in dilated pupils.

Cross cylinder treatment correction divides the cylinder power into two symmetric parts. This astigmatism correction requires less total tissue ablation and preserves the mean corneal radius of curvature, leaving the cornea more prolate and symmetrical with a final shape closer to the normal cornea, while inducing fewer aberrations. The multizone cross-cylinder method also creates a progressive transition, with a low dioptric gradient, between treated and untreated cornea, with the following advantages:

- A physiologically prolate, symmetrical corneal shape.
- Less regression.
- Better visual acuity.
- Increased tissue sparing from the splitting part of cylinder ablation in periphery.

A delicate point in the creation of a new surface with excimer laser ablation is the transition zone (TZ). A marked variation of curvature in the peripheral cornea portion leads to a reduced curvature variation but may induce regression and restriction in the effective optical zone (OZ).

After surgery, we always apply a protective contact lens and give a single administration of cyclopentolate 1% eye drops, preservative-free steroid eye drops, and fluoroquinolone eye drops. The patient is then instructed to use the fluoroquinolone until complete re-epithelialization. We remove the protective contact lens only when the epithelium is completely covering the corneal surface and appears stable. We also prescribe fluorometholone eye drops three times a day for 3 weeks, as well as preservative-free artificial tears six times a day. Postoperative examinations are routinely performed at 1, 3, 6, and 12 months. We do not administer a longer course of steroid because, in our experience, the surface regularity provided by smoothing greatly reduces the postoperative haze and regression.

Detection of residual refractive errors within the first months requires careful topographic examination. Detection of surface irregularity due to the epithelial closure line will be transitory. In case of central topographical irregularities, we apply a soft disposable contact lens for up to 15 days. The pressure applied by the contact lens will typically regularize the epithelium. Detection of frank under-correction should be followed by a course of topical steroid (dexamethasone) eye drops for 1 to 2 weeks with monitoring of intraocular pressure.

Chapter 7

Corneal Biomechanical Effects of Surface Ablation Compared With LASIK Using Microkeratome or Femtosecond Laser

Scipione Rossi, MD

Biomechanical properties of the cornea affect the predictability and stability of refractive surgery outcomes. After different forms of keratorefractive surgery, profound changes in corneal structure and biomechanics may occur, associated with secondary iatrogenic corneal thinning, shape changes, and disruption of collagen lamellar layers.

Corneal Biomechanics

The cornea is not mechanically inert. The biomechanical properties of the cornea affect the predictability and stability of refractive surgery outcomes. The role of corneal biomechanics is important to consider in both routine surface and intrastromal ablation procedures. Biomechanical changes can manifest clinically as immediate corneal shape changes, shape instability over time, and increased sensitivity to shape changes from stimuli such as altered hydration, hypoxia, and subsequent injury or surgery.[1,2] The mechanical response of the cornea to injury is dominated by the *stroma*. On a weight basis, the stroma is approximately 78% water, 15% collagen, and 7% noncollagenous proteins, proteoglycans, and salts. Three hundred to five hundred lamellae run from limbus to limbus and are stacked with angular offsets; this orientation becomes increasingly random in the *anterior stroma* where significantly more oblique branching and interweaving are noted. Interlamellar branching is also more extensive in the *corneal periphery* than in its center. Ultramicroscopy studies and cohesive tensile strength testing showed the stronger, more rigid regions of the cornea were located anteriorly and peripherally.[3]

Interweaving of collagen bundles between neighboring lamellae provides an important structural foundation for shear (sliding) resistance and transfer of tensile loads between lamellae (Figure 7-1).[4]

Corneal Biomechanical Changes After "Surface" and "Intrastromal" Ablation

During keratorefractive surgical procedures involving central ablation, an immediate circumferential severing of corneal lamellae is produced (Figure 7-2). In simple elastic shell models, this results in a forward herniation that, if considered alone, would result in corneal steepening. However, central ablation also relaxes lamellar tension in residual peripheral lamellar segments, which decreases local resistance to

Buratto L, Slade S, Serrao S, Lombardo M. ***PRK: The Past, Present, and Future of Surface Ablation.*** *(pp. 81-84).*

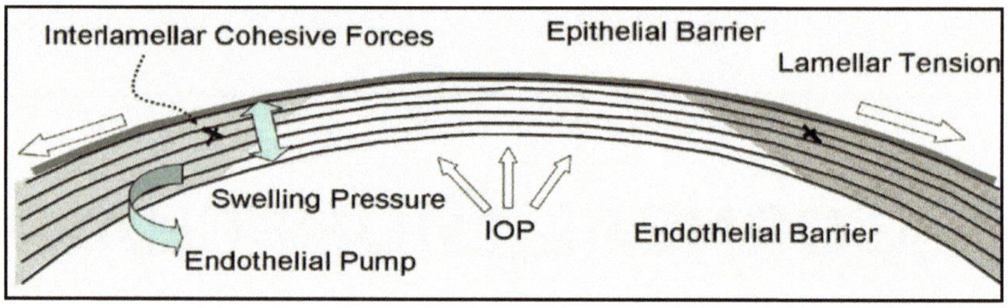

Figure 7-1. Corneal architecture and major biomechanical loading forces in the cornea. Inter-lamellar cohesive forces and collagen interweaving, whose distribution is greater in anterior and peripheral stroma and is indicated by grey shading, provide a means of transmitting centripetal forces to underlying lamellae.[4]

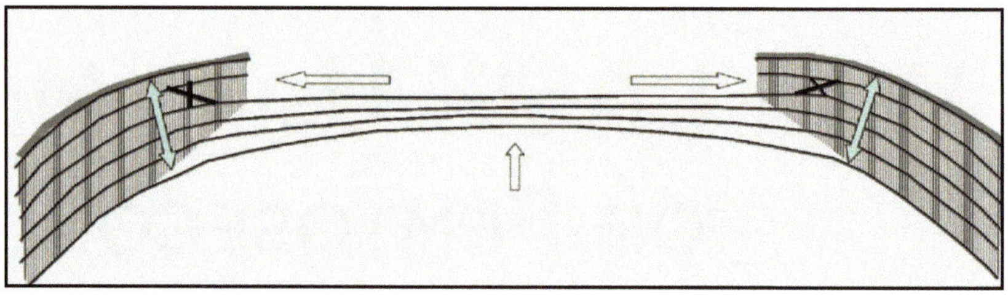

Figure 7-2. A model of biomechanical flattening associated with disruption of central lamellar segments. In this model, we outline a forward movement of posterior corneal surface (fewer collagen cross-links and reduced keratocyte density centrally) and a minor outward movement of peripheral cornea (the limbus doesn't expand).[4]

swelling and results in peripheral stromal thickening.[4] Expansion of the peripheral stroma may generate centripetal stress in underlying lamellae through dense inter-lamellar connections at the margin of the ablation zone. Because the central portions of these lamellae comprise the new anterior surface, there is resulting central flattening.

We know that surface and intra-stromal surgical procedures can affect the biomechanical properties of the cornea, especially when a large amount of laser ablation is required in highly myopic eyes.

Moreover, intra-stromal surgery significantly decreases the corneal biomechanical strength more than surface surgery. This may be due to the fact that LASIK requires both "tissue photo-ablation" and "flap creation," whereas PRK requires "tissue photo-ablation" only. In addition, LASIK also violates the anterior corneal stroma to a deeper level than an equivalent PRK procedure.[5]

Biomechanical Differences in Femtosecond and Microkeratome Corneal Flaps

Femtosecond (FS) laser and mechanical microkeratome (MK) systems have different mechanisms of action to create corneal flaps for LASIK surgery. The mechanical microkeratome uses shearing forces through the use of an oscillating blade travelling across the cornea in a rotational or translational approach. The FS laser is an infrared (1053-nm) laser that creates a corneal resection by delivering ultrafast laser pulses in the 100 fs (100 x 10^{-15} second, 1-µm diameter, which expands to 2 µm to 3 µm) range at a predetermined depth in the cornea. These pulses create micro-photodisruption or an expanding bubble of gas (CO_2) and water that in turn cleave the tissue and create a plane of separation. Pulses are scanned in a spiral or raster pattern and are placed next to each other to create a planar LASIK flap.[6]

The main difference between the FS laser and the MK involves the flap architecture: a planar flap profile for FS laser compared to a meniscus flap profile for MK. A meniscus flap typically extends deeper in the periphery and is shallower in the center of the flap, while a planar flap has a more uniform thickness across its entirety. The use of the FS laser rather than a microkeratome for corneal flap creation determines a better predictability of the flap thickness and guarantees a thinner, uniform, and planar flap, improving the corneal biomechanical stability (Figure 7-3).

Corneal Biomechanical Stability

A thinner flap (90 to 100 µm) produces a corneal loss of strength of 14% compared to a thicker flap (140 to 160 µm) whose loss of strength is about 30% (Figure 7-4).[3]

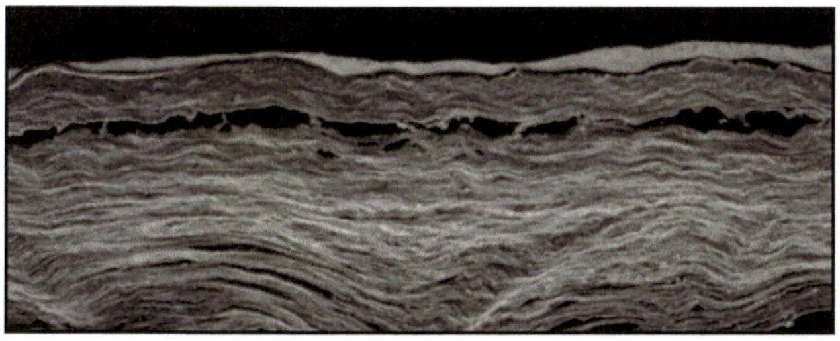

Figure 7-3. Microscopic image of femtosecond LASIK flap.

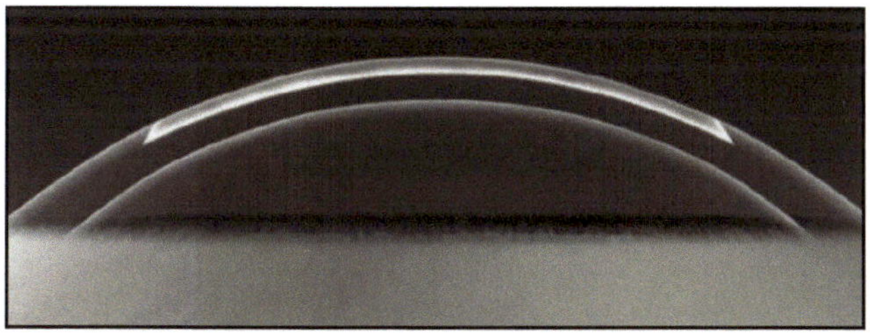

Figure 7-5. 150° inverted bevel-in side-cut performed with the fifth-generation 150-kHz IntraLase femtosecond laser.

The thickness of the post-LASIK stromal bed is critical when LASIK surgery is planned. The prevention of LASIK keratectasia is thought to require at least 250 μm of residual stromal bed (RSB) under the flap.

Another important corneal biomechanical aspect studied by Marshall[3] is that 75% of the weakening in corneal biomechanics in refractive surgery comes from the *side cut*, not from the cuts to the lamellar bed. A 150° bevel in side-cut angle reduces strain change on the cornea (Figure 7-5).

The potential benefits of this side-cut architecture include reduced risk of flap slippage and post- LASIK ectasia by enhancing biomechanical stability. Knorz and Vossmerbaeumer[7] compared a group with 70° cuts to a group with 150° cuts (inverted side-cut) and found that it was 1.5 times harder to dehisce the inverted side-cut group compared with the 70° side-cut group (Figure 7-6).

In conclusion, several factors such as flap diameter, method of construction, thickness, and flap side-cut angle all affect the biomechanical properties of the post-operative LASIK cornea. Fortunately, these often can be adjusted to improve the stability and optics of the eye.

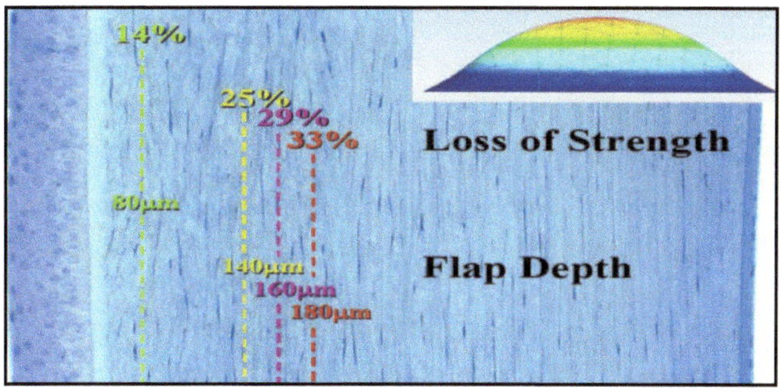

Figure 7-4. Correlation between corneal loss of strength and flap thickness.[3]

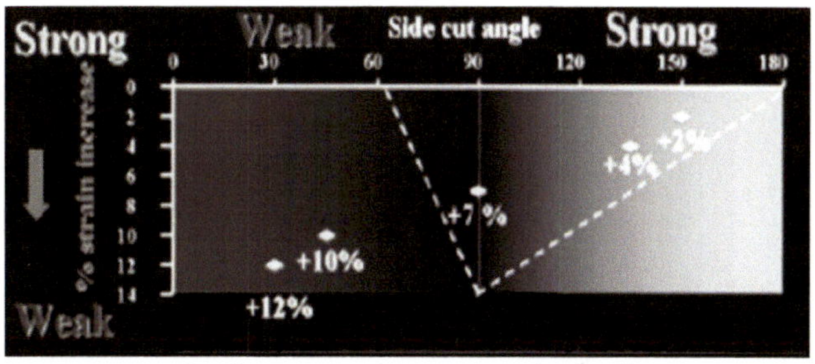

Figure 7-6. The image assigns numerical values to strain distribution, showing that a bevel-in side-cut results in very little increase in strain, whereas vertical and bevel-out side-cut angles increase strain.

References

1. Roberts C. Biomechanics of the cornea and wavefront-guided laser refractive surgery. *J Refract Surg.* 2002;18:S589-S592.
2. Netto MV, Wilson SE. Corneal wound healing relevance to wavefront guided laser treatments. *Ophthalmol Clin North Am.* 2004;17:225-231.
3. Marshall J. Sub-Bowman's keratomileusis (SBK) vs. PRK. Presented at 11th ESCRS Winter Refractive Meeting; Athens, 2007.
4. Dupps WJ Jr, Roberts C. Effect of acute biomechanical changes on corneal curvature after photokeratectomy. *J Refract Surg.* 2001;17:658-669.
5. Khoramnia R, Lohmann CP, Wuellner C, et al. Effect of 3 excimer laser ablation frequencies (200 Hz, 500Hz, 1000Hz) on the cornea using a 1000Hz scanning-spot excimer laser. *J Cataract Refract Surg.* 2010;36:1385-1391.
6. Slade SG. The use of femtosecond laser in the customization of corneal flaps in laser in situ keratomileusis. *Curr Opin Ophthalmol.* 2007;18:314-317.
7. Knorz MC, Vossmerbaeumer U. Comparison of flap adhesion strength using the Amadeus microkeratome and the IntraLase iFS femtosecond laser in rabbits. *J Refract Surg.* 2008;24:875-878.

Chapter 8

The Athens Protocol PRK and CXL

Anastasios John Kanellopoulos, MD

A second procedure for visual rehabilitation may sometimes be needed after cornea collagen cross-linking (CXL) for treatment of progressive keratoconus or post-LASIK ectasia. Following many years of employing CXL for ectasia cases, we introduced the "Athens protocol": same-day topography-guided partial PRK and CXL.

Our findings support that simultaneous topography-guided partial PRK with CXL offers a safe and effective approach for normalizing the cornea and enhancing visual function in eyes with ectatic conditions. The core importance of combining CXL in this technique is to address highly irregular astigmatism in the management of eyes with keratoconus and post-LASIK ectasia.

Our theoretical and clinical evidence supports the use of this "Athens protocol" where CXL and topography-guided surface ablation are performed in the same session rather than sequentially over time.

It is our experience that surface ablation using the topography-guided excimer laser platform (Allegretto, Alcon/WaveLight) effectively and predictably normalizes the corneal surface and improves functional vision, and we believe there is a synergistic effect when this procedure is performed simultaneously with CXL.

Safety with our combination approach has been favorable as well. Although postoperative haze and delayed epithelial healing have occurred, these have been minor complications in a small number of eyes within our large series. Out of the 400 eyes studied, just two required repeat CXL, and none needed to have a cornea transplant.

Meeting Visual Rehabilitation Needs

Although the efficacy of CXL for stabilizing keratectasia is well-established and the procedure also causes some corneal flattening, significant residual astigmatism limiting contact lens wear may be a persistent problem for some patients. This situation creates an indication to perform topography-guided PRK.

While surface ablation in a keratoconic eye may sound unorthodox, the goal of our treatment using the topography-guided software is to normalize the corneal surface and improve best-corrected acuity. This is a therapeutic procedure, not a refractive one. In fact, some eyes turn out more myopic postoperatively, but have significant regularity and best spectacle-corrected visual acuity. We use surface ablation to remove no more than 50 µm of stroma and typically treat only 2 to 2.5 D of astigmatism and up to 1 D of myopia.

Buratto L, Slade S, Serrao S, Lombardo M. *PRK: The Past, Present, and Future of Surface Ablation.* (pp. 85-88).

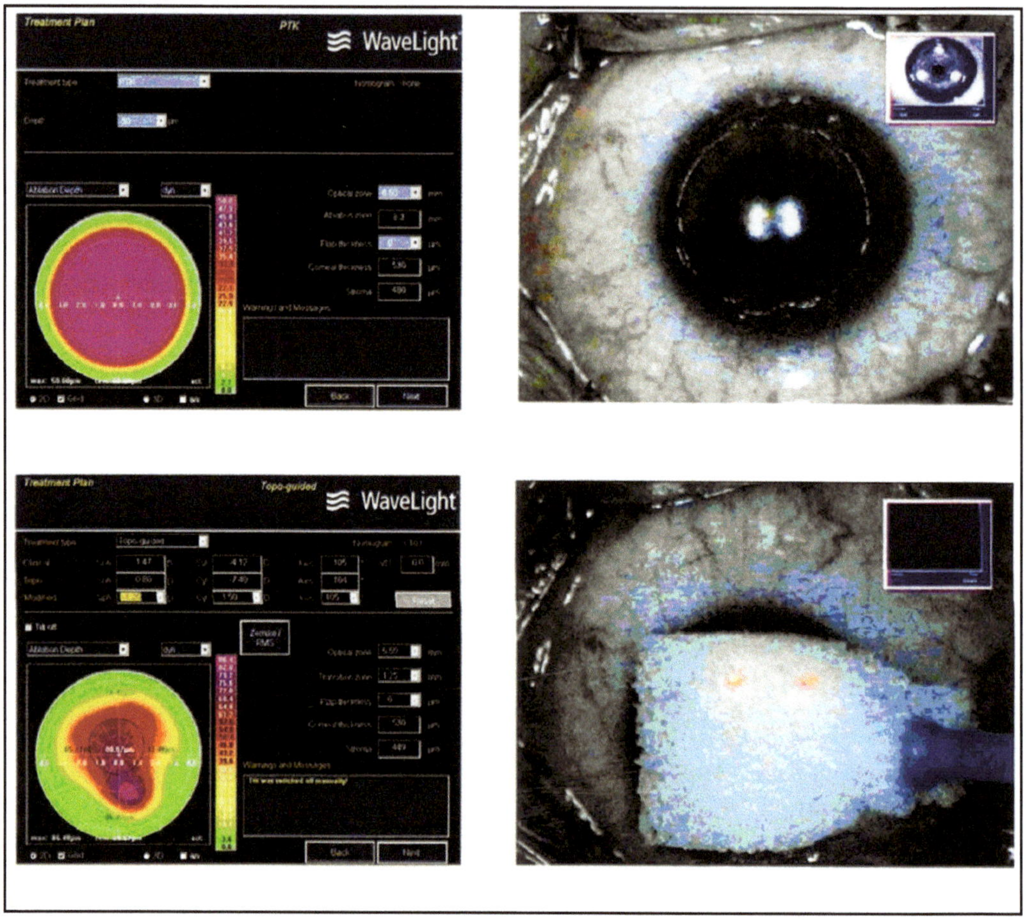

Figure 8-1. The basic steps of the Athens Protocol: Top left, The PTK treatment is planned on the Alcon/WaveLight platform. Top right, Following the PTK, areas of Bowman's have been ablated by the PTK, confirming that the epithelium over the cone is thinner. Bottom left, The treatment plans of the topography-guided partial PRK that is the core concept of this protocol. Bottom right, MC application prior to the riboflavin and CXL.

The protocol begins with a 6.5-mm phototherapeutic keratectomy (PTK) to remove 50 µm of epithelium. Then, the topography-guided partial PRK is performed followed by mitomycin C application (0.02% for 20 seconds) and the CXL procedure. The excimer laser ablation resembles part of a hyperopic treatment. It is performed using a 5.5-mm effective optical zone and targets steepening of the area adjacent to the cone in an attempt to regularize the corneal surface (Figure 8-1).

We believe our rationale for performing the two procedures simultaneously with the ablation first has several advantages. We have reported data showing that the corneal epithelium and Bowman's membrane can act as barriers to UVA light penetration into the stroma. As these tissues are removed with the PTK/PRK procedure, it seems intuitive that the efficacy of the CXL procedure would be increased. This concept is supported by clinical findings outlined below.

For example, in a patient who had CXL alone in one eye and the Athens protocol in the other, inspection of OCT maps for hyper-reflectivity, which we recently described as a sign of the extent of cross-linking, shows the area of cross-linking is much broader and denser in the latter eye.

We additionally introduced the theory that the PRK-treated eye represents a better biomechanical model for performing the CXL procedure. In theory, an eye with a more regularized surface from CXL as opposed to an irregular untreated cornea would be better able to handle ongoing strain from IOP and eye rubbing over the cone peak and would more likely remain more stable.

We believe redistribution of corneal strain by remodeling the cornea with surface ablation is a significant factor in the synergistic effect achieved when performing the two procedures together. The simultaneous procedure also avoids removing cross-linked cornea, which occurs when performing CXL first followed by the laser treatment.

Results from a comparison of two large, consecutive series of eyes treated at the same session or with CXL first followed 1 year later by a topography-guided surface ablation showed statistically significant differences in a number of outcome parameters favoring the same-day procedure. The study, which

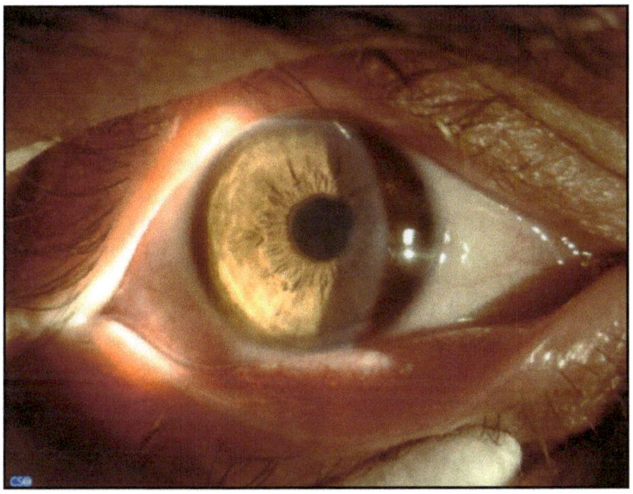

Figure 8-2. A clinical picture of the right eye of a 27-year-old man with advanced KCN. Preop BSCVA was 20/50 with -2.5 -5 @80. The patient underwent the Athens Protocol and is now UCVA 20/30 and BSCVA 20/20 with -1 -1.5 @85. The slit-lamp photo shows the corneal clarity and the ground-glass appearance typical of CXL.

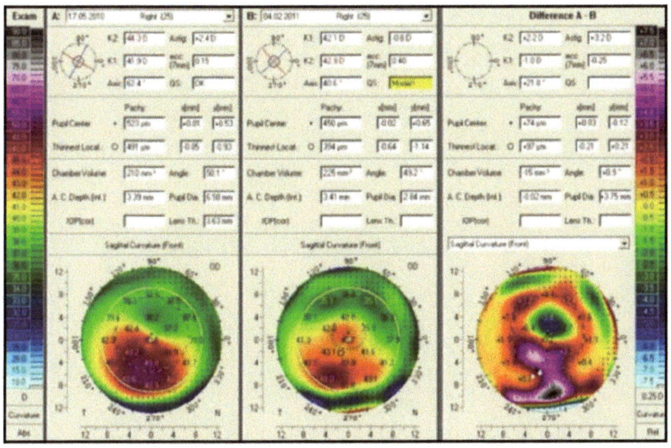

Figure 8-4. A comparison of preoperative and 7 months postoperative of Pentacam images showing the significant normalization of the cone and keratometric flattening and better symmetry.

has been published,[1] included 127 eyes in the sequential group and 198 eyes treated with the Athens protocol (Figure 8-2).

For the eyes in the sequential group, mean logMAR uncorrected visual acuity (UCVA) improved from 0.9 to 0.49, mean logMAR best spectacle-corrected visual acuity improved from 0.41 to 0.16, mean K decreased by 2.75 D and mean MRSE by 2.5 D, and the mean haze score was 1.2. For the eyes in the simultaneous group, there was a significantly greater improvement in mean logMAR UCVA (from 0.96 to 0.3) and mean logMAR BSCVA (from 0.39 to 0.11) as well as a significantly greater mean reduction in MRSE (-3.2 D)

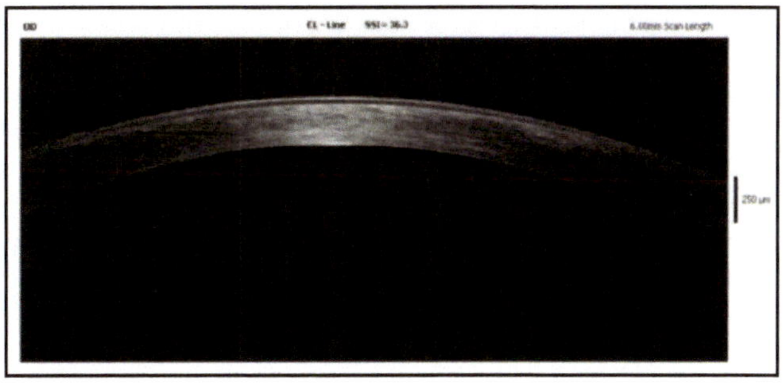

Figure 8-3. Cornea OCT of the same eye 7 months postop Athens Protocol. One can appreciate the anterior cornea hyper-reflectivity consistent with CXL and the demarcation line at about 300 μm depth depicting (as we have introduced and published) the depth of effective CXL. Those clinicians familiar with findings following CXL alone may appreciate the enhanced depth and diameter of the CXL effect noted on OCT supporting the advantage on the eye with the Athens Protocol.

and keratometry (-3.5 D) (Figures 8-3 and 8-4). The mean haze score in the simultaneous group was 0.5, and that was significantly lower than in the controls. Central corneal thickness decreased by 70 µm after both procedures, and there was no significant change in endothelial cell count in either group. These findings demonstrate that performing the two procedures together offers advantages of less PRK-associated scarring and better riboflavin and UVA penetration to achieve a wider and deeper CXL effect with greater corneal flattening.

Reference

1. Kanellopoulos AJ. Comparison of sequential vs same-day simultaneous collagen cross-linking and topography-guided PRK for treatment of keratoconus. *J Refract Surg.* 2009;25(9):S812-S818.

Bibliography

Kanellopoulos AJ. Cross-linking plus topography-guided PRK for post-LASIK Ectasia Management. In: Garg A, Rosen E, eds. *Instant Clinical Diagnosis in Ophthalmology Refractive Surgery.* New Delhi, India: Jaypee Brothers; 2008:258-269.

Kanellopoulos AJ. Cross-linking plus topography-guided PRK for post-LASIK ectasia management. In: Garg A, ed. *Mastering Advanced Surface Ablation Techniques.* New Delhi, India: Jaypee Brothers; 2007:204-214.

Kanellopoulos AJ. Cross-linking plus topography-guided PRK for post-LASIK ectasia management. In: Garg A, Pinelli R, Brart DO, Lovisolo CF, eds. *Mastering Corneal Collagen Cross-linking Techniques (C3-CCL/CxL) with Video DVD Rom.* New Delhi, India: Jaypee Brothers; 2008:69-80.

Kanellopoulos AJ. Crystalens HD: the accommodative IOL technique. In: Garg A, Alio JL, eds. *Surgical Techniques in Ophthalmology: Refractive Surgery.* New Delhi, India: Jaypee-Highlights; 2009:301-304.

Kanellopoulos AJ. In-flap simultaneous collagen crosslinking (CXL) and topography-guided (tPRK) for early Post-LASIK ectasia: a novel technique. In: Garg A, Alio JL, eds. *Surgical Techniques in Ophthalmology: Refractive Surgery.* New Delhi, India: Jaypee-Highlights; 2009:233-236.

Kanellopoulos AJ. Intralase-assisted LASIK, video V; Comparison of topography guided to standard LASIK for hyperopia, video VI; Limited topoguided PRK followed by collagen cross linking for keratoconus, video VII. In: Garg A, ed. *Video Atlas of Ophthalmic Surgery.* New Delhi, India: Jaypee Brothers; 2007

Kanellopoulos AJ. PRK and C3-R. In: Boxer Wachler BS, ed. *Modern Management of Keratoconus.* New Delhi, India: Jaypee Brothers; 2007:219-228.

Kanellopoulos AJ. Prophylactic collagen crosslinking in high risk femtosecond assisted-LASIK: a novel technique. In: Garg A, Alio JL, eds. *Surgical Techniques in Ophthalmology: Refractive Surgery.* New Delhi, India: Jaypee-Highlights; 2009:423-426.

Kanellopoulos AJ. Simultaneous prophylactic collagen cross-linking (CXL) following high-risk topography-guided PRK (tPRK). In: Garg A, Alio JL, eds. *Surgical Techniques in Ophthalmology: Refractive Surgery.* New Delhi, India: Jaypee-Highlights; 2009:427-430.

Kanellopoulos AJ. Simultaneous collagen cross-linking (CXL) and topography-guided PRK (tPRK) for keratoconus (KCN). In: Garg A, Alio JL, eds. *Surgical Techniques in Ophthalmology: Refractive Surgery.* New Delhi, India: Jaypee-Highlights; 2009:18-21.

Kanellopoulos AJ. Simultaneous collagen crosslinking (CXL) and topography-guided PRK (tPRK) for keratoconus (KCN). In: Garg A, Alio JL, eds. *Surgical Techniques in Ophthalmology: Refractive Surgery.* New Delhi, India: Jaypee-Highlights; 2009:60-63.

Chapter 9

Surface Ablation (PRK) to Enhance Previous LASIK

William Trattler, MD and David A. Goldman, MD

For the past 15 years, LASIK has been a popular procedure for correcting myopia, hyperopia, and astigmatism. Although LASIK typically provides very accurate visual results, a small percentage of patients will require enhancements shortly after their procedure. As time passes, a small percentage of patients may experience a refractive shift, requiring further laser vision correction. Although some surgeons prefer lifting LASIK flaps for enhancements, there are risks to this technique, including epithelial ingrowth and flap striae. As well, by ablating the previously untouched stroma under the flap, the risk of symptomatic dryness and ectasia may also increase. The alternative procedure, surface ablation over flaps, has proven to be a very effective technique in our experience. This article will discuss the indications and steps to optimize this procedure.

Patient selection is critical for effectively providing laser vision correction enhancements. Evaluation of the ocular surface for dry eye and blepharitis is required, and these conditions must be treated prior to proceeding to enhancements. Evaluation of the individual LASIK flap itself is also important. This includes identifying the location of the flap hinge as well as noting whether there are microstriae present. Corneal topography is a critical tool, as patients with regular or irregular astigmatism should be carefully evaluated to ensure that they do not have early ectasia. Manifest refraction is required to ensure the patient is correctable to 20/20 and, if not, to determine the underlying reason. Cycloplegic refractions should also be performed to determine any latent refractive error. Wavefront testing is also useful, to both measure higher-order aberrations as well as a potential method to drive the laser treatment. Posterior float measurements, as tested by scanning slit-lamps such as the Orbscan (Bausch + Lomb), can be greatly affected by previous LASIK and are not necessary for preoperative evaluation.

Once the preoperative assessment has been completed and the patient has been educated on the risks, benefits, and alternatives to surface ablation, the patient can be prepared for treatment. The surgeon will decide whether to perform alcohol-assisted PRK, LASEK, manual epithelial removal with a blade, epi-LASIK, or laser epithelial removal. Although some surgeons may consider epithelial removal with the Amoils brush, this technique has an increased risk of flap dislocation, in our opinion, and will not be discussed in this chapter. Epi-LASIK, as well, poses the risk of flap dislocation and/or stromal incursions and will be omitted.

For alcohol-assisted PRK or LASEK, surgeons can use either sterile ethanol or isopropyl alcohol, which can be diluted and safely applied. Because there is a small risk of flap dislocation if the epithelium is

Buratto L, Slade S, Serrao S, Lombardo M. *PRK: The Past, Present, and Future of Surface Ablation.* (pp. 89-90).

adherent, we recommend applying the dilute alcohol for an extra 10 to 20 seconds. This allows the epithelium to be removed more easily. Care should be taken to manipulate and slide the epithelium away from the LASIK hinge, as this provides traction to the flap and helps prevent a flap dislocation. Removal of the epithelium should also begin well within the borders of the original LASIK flap to minimize the chance of lifting the flap. With manual epithelial removal, it is even more critical to carefully slide the epithelium in the direction away from the hinge.

Once the epithelium has been removed, the underlying stroma will be visible. It is common to see microstriae (Figure 9-1). In many cases, the standard laser ablation will slightly smooth these striae. However, in cases of severe striae, a very superficial PTK may be advisable. If a PTK is performed, then a surgeon should avoid a wavefront-guided ablation and should instead provide an ablation based on the refraction. Because removing the striae may affect the final refractive outcome, caution should be taken with the amount of refractive error that will be attempted. In some cases, it may be most prudent to only perform the PTK and return 2 to 3 months later for a final surface laser enhancement of the residual refractive error. However, if PRK is performed following PTK, it is important to take into account any hyperopic shift the PTK may induce.

Mitomycin C 0.02% application is an important step. Although the risk of haze is low with surface ablation to enhance previous LASIK, we believe the risk of haze is higher than in virgin corneas. Therefore, MMC is an important safety step. We typically recommend 10 to 20 seconds of MMC application. However, in patients who have high levels of UV exposure (lifeguards, boaters, etc), a longer application time of MMC may be prudent.

Following the procedure, we recommend specific postoperative medications. Topical steroids are particularly important, as unchecked inflammation can lead to diffuse lamellar keratitis (DLK). As well, it is important to check the intraocular pressure during the postoperative period carefully, as rarely a patient can experience elevated IOP and develop diffuse interstitial stromal keratitis (DISK). Broad-spectrum antibiotics, such as the fourth-generation fluoroquinolones, should also be used to minimize risk of infection. Optimizing the ocular surface is also important to speed epithelial healing, and topical medications such as cyclosporine and azithromycin should be initiated prior to any refractive procedure if necessary.

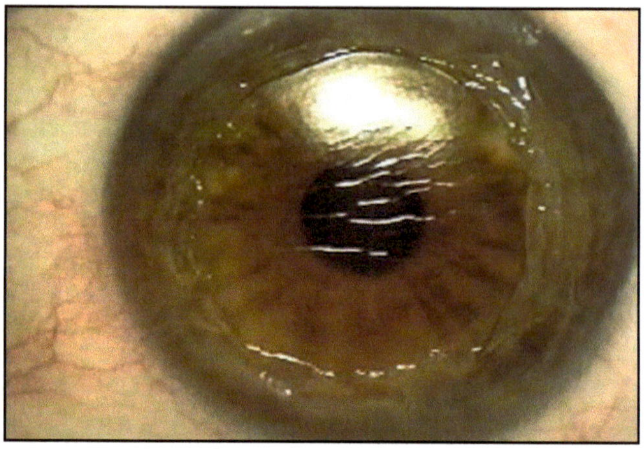

Figure 9-1. Photo of a patient who underwent PRK following LASIK with visible microstriae.

Conclusion

Surface ablation to enhance previous LASIK is a safe and effective procedure for patients who develop residual refractive error. The procedure has the potential benefits of reducing epithelial ingrowth and effectively treating refractive errors. Conventional, topo-guided, and wavefront-guided ablations can be employed, and most patients will experience very good visual results. Finally, prevention of haze and optimizing the ocular surface are two important steps for ensuring the best results with this procedure.

Financial Disclosures

Elena Albé, MD has no financial or proprietary interest in the materials presented herein.

Waleed A. Allam, MD, PhD has no financial or proprietary interest in the materials presented herein.

Lucio Buratto, MD had research and reviewer support, travel expenses, indirect donation or provision of equipment with Alcon, Amo, B+L, Zeiss, STAAR, Technolas, Hoya, and OO Group Medicongress.

David A. Goldman, MD is a consultant to Alcon, Allergan, and Bausch + Lomb.

Anastasios John Kanellopoulos, MD is a consultant for Alcon WaveLight.

Mounir A. Khalifa, MD, PhD is a consultant for Alcon WaveLight, and recieved a research grant from AMO.

Marco Lombardo, MD, PhD has not disclosed any relevant financial relationships.

Scipione Rossi, MD has not disclosed any relevant financial relationships.

Sebastiano Serrao, MD, PhD has not disclosed any relevant financial relationships.

Stephen G. Slade, MD, FACS has not disclosed any relevant financial relationships.

William Trattler, MD is a consultant for and received research support from Abbott Medical Optics, Allergan, and Merck.

Paolo Vinciguerra, MD is a consultant for NIDEK and OCULUS.

R. Vinciguerra, MD has not disclosed any relevant financial relationships.

Index